Mr. Beauty

AN AFFAIR WITH THE BEAUTY INDUSTRY

Robert Montagnese

Cover design by Clea Conner Chang

ISBN: 1508619573
ISBN 13: 9781508619574
Library of Congress Control Number: 2015903160
Createspace Independent Publishing Platform
North Charleston, South Carolina

For Eileen McKenna
Colleague and Friend

Acknowledgements

I n the stretch for dreams there are those who are there to provide a leg up. Thank you John Higgins for your support and love. Thank you Maryanne Delaney Martin for your guidance in the development of this book and Clea and Jonathan Chang for the many creative insights you provided. Finally, my deepest appreciation for all the women willing to spend their time, and share personal thoughts on the topic of beauty.

Table of Contents

Pucker Up

Observation is key to understanding beauty. Actually, it is the key to understanding life.

Early one morning I was on the #1 train traveling south when I noticed a woman seated in front of me applying lipstick. The rest of her was already made up with jungle red nails, a warm tone foundation and lengthening mascara. The lipstick was the final touch. It always is. As the train moved along she maneuvered with great artistry not to mention dexterity. When she looked up at me I smiled and she went back to her ritual. Once done, she looked back up at me and this time smiled backed. The woman seated to her right noticed it and then smiled at both of us. Interestingly, it was the nod of approval from the woman seated next to her, not mine, that resulted in a delighted expression on her face.

Kaput

had been recruited back to an advertising agency to correct a poor client relationship and creative issues that were ongoing for some time. It was familiar territory for me as I had left the company only five years earlier to work for the beauty competition. This had been my third return, but that is a story for another time. Once the offer for my return was final, I asked the person responsible for the transition what should I tell my current boss, that is, the reason for my abrupt resignation. She said with a grin, "Tell them that you were on borrowed time." And there I went to save the day greeted with much fanfare and welcome. Almost five years into my return it all started to unravel.

Much of the tailspin was the result of ignorance and ended in arrogance. I should have allowed my instinct to serve me better as the changes on both client and agency side made it obvious that old relationships were no longer valued. New loyalties were being established. There was a time in the industry when brand knowledge and insight had greater value. This currency provided a level of continuity that nurtured the brand equity, however, it was a new generation.

I am afraid that today with the proliferation of media and messages, brand value is driven by instant gratification and short-term gains. In essence there is very little loyalty that remains for most brands, more unfortunately, most people.

The disruption of my career was a year in the making, but it took a cheap leather - or perhaps vinyl bag - being tossed at me from the driveway of the Chateau Marmont in LA to end the entire ordeal.

I surmised her behavior had something to do with a plethora of panic emails from that morning. It wasn't even 8AM, and the streams of emails were already out of control in regard to a commercial that was in postproduction and running behind schedule. I had managed a number of these delays in the past and thought with a bit of planning we would be able to make up lost time. I am a former O.R. nurse who was quick with a clamp in the operating suite. After all, these things happened all the time in the business of making lipstick commercials and to keep it in perspective, we were not late in getting a lung delivered to a waiting recipient! I was told that I underestimated the gravity of the situation. The flinging bag, leather or not, was her non-verbal hostile reaction to the morning news.

We were on our way to a photo shoot for a very blond rock star. It began in an SUV on our way to the set. I believe the words I used were something like "aggressive and unnecessary behavior". My team sat in horrified silence behind me knowing that I was brave in confronting what were months of verbal abuse. I do maintain that ambition at a certain age is unattractive no matter what the situation.

Arriving at the photo shoot with the mad lady in tow she exited the SUV and announced to anyone who would listen that she was wearing her "rock star" outfit. Do people still consider having east and west coast outfits other than taking into consideration the change in temperature? I remember a former client from the mid-west telling me about her New York City "power suit", but that was sometime back in the mid-eighties. We are now talking many years later but still I never forgot it.

I managed to slip into the studio where the shoot was taking place to find an empty chair at a folding table. In the past I would have been escorted to the talent's dressing room for a hello and kiss-kiss on both cheeks (above the waist that is - although in this business it may as well be the other). There, in a dirty studio off of Sunset Boulevard, it was her show and I was relegated to a room away from the action and intentionally out of sight. I settled into my chair, took a deep breath, and said to myself "mortgage payments".

Looking back now I remember very little about the rock star photo shoot itself. Maybe because it was just one more in a thousand or so that had come before it - with products, props and people on all sides all playing the same redundant roles.

To add to the imposed isolation of that day, probably the result of the morning conflict, I learned by reading a long email trail from the client to the "bag lady" that we, the agency, were not allowed to stay at the same hotel as they the client, but she, of course, was an exception to the rule. Oh yes, the art of team building gone wrong in LA.

During the next couple of rainy days in LA there were two phones calls that changed the course of things. The first was to my partner back in New York. The second call was to Human Resource to resign (to the same person who wooed me almost five years earlier). What I learned on that fateful trip was that not only is aggressive behavior at a particular age unattractive but also, and even more so, was the negative impact of self-importance on others. My team was beginning to leave the agency one by one.

Bare Feet Tuna

F ast forward. I had served the mandated time at the agency in order to secure my exit package. I was now standing at the black marble counter top in the kitchen of my country house in bare feet, wearing only a pair of navy blue nylon gym shorts, making a tuna salad sandwich. While neatly chopping a red onion, through the din echoed an advertisement for Avon. It caught my attention. I put the knife down and turned up the volume.

At the time I called it a sabbatical, but the fact was I left a very lucrative position in a large advertising agency that spring. Leaving, I tried to convince myself it was a good thing and would rationalize it in many ways; some of which were at the very least entertaining. The truth is I was pushed out. The new power players put in charge operated partly in fear, partly in ignorance. Change on the account was inevitable. While change was part of this evolution, strong leadership should have remained a constant. It was not.

I was now living one hundred miles from the city, in "the country" (as we like to call it) making tuna salad sandwiches standing in my bare feet. While I was spending my summer in this quiet spot I had a lot of time to dissect the situation that lead me there, as well, aspects of a lifetime in beauty advertising. Working on some writing and practicing piano provided some diversion; let's say "filling time" during my day. But there was very little that could distract me from the annoying voice in my head asking over and over if at age fifty-six would I ever get another chance.

Moving closer towards the television I sensed the voice coming from the monitor was speaking directly to me. The voice over talent with a smooth but exuberant tone (good casting, I thought) was channeling this message to me "How would you like to be an Avon sales representative?" Instantaneously I knew the annoying repetitive voice in my head had been answered. Without finishing the tuna salad I went directly to my computer, closed out of LinkedIn (the pseudo career lifeline), and googled "Avon Representative". The closest office to my Upper West Side apartment in the city was in East Harlem. I cancelled my plans for the following day and scheduled my interview with Avon completely optimistic that I would get another chance.

Ding Dong

was to meet the District Manager at ten o'clock in the morning. I took the M116 bus crosstown then up to 116th street. This was an area with which I was not very familiar. When I got off the bus I began walking north on Frederick Douglas Boulevard. I was about two blocks from my destination when I realized that I was about to go into a meeting without a pen and pad in hand. Fortunately, I spotted a Duane Reade across the street. I stepped into the store and found what I needed. In my excitement, I almost told the check out lady why I needed them but decided that might be a bit weird. At the corner I saw the sign in the window "Avon East Harlem District Office". It wasn't a big corporate logo kind of sign rather a simple paper banner that was in the window.

Over the years I have been in meetings with the CEO's and presidents of Proctor & Gamble, L'Oreal, Coca-Cola, Miles Laboratories, Nespresso, Kohl's and JC Penney just to name a few. I've attended the Golden Globes, Academy Awards, SAG Awards, Grammy's, MTV Awards and Tony's multiple times. During that time I've had the pleasure of meeting people like Princess Diana, and Brook Astor and even have had lunch with Diane Keaton at the Polo Lounge in Beverly Hills. I've had tea with Jennifer Lopez and Arlene (her best friend at the time) at the Oak Room in the Plaza Hotel in New York just before she was to become the superstar she is today.

There were drinks with Jennifer Aniston at the Sunset Towers in Los Angeles and dinner with Andie MacDowell at Joe Allen's on Restaurant Row. Then there was the time I was sent out to woo talent like Charleze Theron over coffee at the Chateau Marmont in LA. I had drinks with Lance Armstrong, who said he would never endorse a hair color product for men and breakfast with a very young and sweet Jennifer Love Hewitt and her mother.

Adding to this roster of celebrity were artists which included the legendary Vidal Sassoon; the shy, considerate genius Kevin Aucoin; the brilliant Mathew Rolston; the revolutionary Peggy Sirota; the visionary Mario Testino; the masterful Kenneth Willardt; the sensitive Pierluca de Carlo; the dynamic Laurent Chanez, and on and on. All of whom I was fortunate enough to work with over the years.

There were the numerous luncheons with editors, including Anna, Glenda, Kate; and publishers, the likes of the dynamic Donna, Agnes and Jill. Many of them referred to me as "Mr. Beauty". With all of that under my belt I still felt a bit unnerved by what I was about to do. I stopped in front of the door leading into the East Harlem District office and took a deep breath thinking to myself—I'm about to become an Avon Lady.

I found the Harlem office as inviting as a temporary election campaign headquarters. Inside there were folding tables with chairs and posters. Products, dolls, boxes and piles of pamphlets were all over the place. The view from inside looking out was blocked by posters that were in place using double stick tape. On the interior the walls were covered with visuals of Reese Witherspoon, and Fergie (with whom I had the loveliest exchange at the "Night Before Party" for the Oscars along with Tom Hanks and the beautiful Rita Wilson—who thought that I was someone she knew). Interspersed between the two celebrities were additional posters of everyday women with captions printed below their faces that said, "Believe in your own Success" and "Say Hello to a New Tomorrow". After reading them, I felt comforted that I made a good choice. I was greeted, told to take a seat and asked if I would like coffee all in one breath.

Once the coffee was on the table (served not in Limoges china, but in Styrofoam cups), Genevieve, the District Manager, dressed in a floral cotton dress that accented her round shape, took a seat opposite me and smiled. I returned a smile and then opened my new note pad, creasing the perfectly smooth cover to the first page which was very white and ready to be used to capture all the information that I was about to receive. I was also hoping that Genevieve got the impression that I was prepared and serious about this. She proceeded to ask me a variety of questions ranging from the origin of my last name and my place of birth, to what I have been doing lately. I responded quickly and at times cryptically about my professional background only giving her enough to feel comfortable that I wasn't some kind of pervert. I sensed that she liked me so much that I felt like I was sitting with one of my Italian aunts talking in her kitchen;

the scent of a pot of gravy simmering on the stove wafting across the room.

After the initial personal information was recorded-address, numbers, etcetera - Genevieve got up from the table and went to a shelf behind her to get the "Global Appointment Kit" from the wall of kits stacked in the corner. She selected one under a cardboard sign that read "English" rather than the wall with the sign indicating "Spanish". I noticed when she placed it on the table there were numbers printed on the package. It was number 3463040. I immediately wondered if it was an indication of how many kits Genevieve has passed out in her lifetime at Avon. It wouldn't surprise me given how energetic she appeared to be from the moment I met her. She sat back down at the table with her hands resting on the kit almost as if she was protecting a file from the *Da Vinci Code* containing top-secret information. Before she opened it Genevieve leaned forward and in a low whisper said, "Let's talk".

When she turned the first page of the "Say Hello to a New Tomorrow" brochure, she began her pitch. I already knew about the huge empowerment factor that is a large part of Avon's brand equity. At the time of my interview, Avon was the number two beauty company globally. The door-to-door sales force contributing to this success numbered six million plus women around the world. The company provides all women the opportunity to make a living. The flexibility of a sales position with Avon is attractive to many - especially women who are not interested in working in a structured office environment or are lacking the skills to do so. Others are not able to be away from home for long periods of time. Still there are those who live in rural areas where employment opportunities are few and far between. The corporate mantra of "a company of women for women" underscores a support system that assists any woman interested in tips on effective selling techniques, product education and incentives to earn more money and ultimately, a sense of recognition. Hearing about these elements face to face with Genevieve was inspirational. Even as a jaded beauty junkie I was ready to sign up!

When Genevieve turned to the next page there was a black and white photo of Andrea Jung, Avon's CEO. She was seated on a wooden stool wearing her signature oversized pearl choker. Genevieve pointed to the photo and with reverence told me who it was. Andrea was the Chairman and Chief Executive Officer of the company. If I managed to sell $112,000 worth of Avon products, I might be able to meet her in Alaska at the President's Club celebration. I didn't have the heart to tell Genevieve that I had already met Andrea twice. Her step-nephew, by a former marriage, was once an intern working for me. I never sold the required quota to win the trip to Alaska. I imagine Andrea and her signature pearl choker never made it either. Six months after my meeting with Genevieve, Andrea was being replaced as the CEO at Avon.

Our meeting continued and I was fascinated by many of the things I was learning about Avon. The first is that a man named David H. McConnell founded the company in 1886. Back then the company was called the California Perfume Company. In 1926 the company took on the new name Avon, inspired by McConnell's travel to Stratford-on-Avon, England. He started out selling books and early on recognized that most of his potential customers were women. He used sample bottles of perfume he made as an incentive for their time. He quickly realized that the women he met were far more interested in the perfume than the books. Mr. McConnell also observed during this time that the women he met had a need to help with the household expenses and thought they would be a perfect choice for selling perfume to other women.

A woman by the name of Mrs. P. F. E. Albee was chosen by Mr. McConnell to be the first sales representative for Avon. She was from New Hampshire and at the age of 50 would travel by horse and buggy or train, depending on distance, to sell the various perfumes door to door. Mr. McConnell referred to her as the "Mother of the California Perfume Company". I learned that she told Mr. McConnell that as a sales representative for his company she thought his perfume provided a lucrative opportunity that was both "pleasant and satisfactory". Because she set a standard of professional behavior in the early years at the company, Mrs. Albee is still remembered at Avon after one hundred and twenty-five years. Every year an exclusive Mrs. Albee doll, which resembles a Gibson Girl, is designed as an award for superior sales results. I did notice a number of porcelain dolls standing on a shelf in Genevieve's district office marking her achievements.

During the hour or so that I was there I was inundated with reading materials, selling tip brochures, incentive plans to earn more, product samples, mini skin care flip chart booklets and shade color chips for lips and nails. Before our conversation ended I was asked to make a list, with Genevieve's watchful eye focusing on the page upon which I wrote, of the first fifty women that I would contact. Of course, none of them were celebrities.

Corner to Corner

left the Avon office and began to walk south to 116th Street to the bus stop. The experience that I had just had was exhilarating. I felt inspired thinking about all the possibilities in exploring beauty. When I got to the corner I stopped and took a picture with my Blackberry of me and my Avon complimentary tote bag that contained my new world. With a Mary Tyler Moore smile on my face I clicked the picture of me with the bag hanging on the fence behind me in frame. Just then the plastic strap on my Avon tote bag broke, resulting in a display of cosmetics, pamphlets, charts, order forms, and skin creams spewed out across the sidewalk. Was it an omen? I gathered it all up and with one of the two straps still intact, I tied it around the top of the bag and now held it in my arms like a bag of groceries while I waited for the bus. Crossing town I stared out the window thinking about the adventure that was about to begin.

I do my best thinking staring out windows and, in my career I had some beautiful views to stare out at. Take my first corner office at 385 Lexington. It was a modest office building, but the corner office on the fifteenth floor looked towards the Empire State Building, the aorta of New York City. The corner office after that was further up north, 750 Third Avenue to be exact. I don't remember the floor but it was higher than the one on Lexington and I still had my view of the Empire State building and the floor was high enough to clear midtown. I could see all the way west to the Hudson River. Following that panoramic view was my corner office at 777 Third Avenue, only a few blocks north of the previous one and this time facing east. From this office, on a floor higher then the last, I could see the East River and all the way over to Long Island City and the iconic Pepsi sign. The last corner office I occupied was at 622 Third Avenue. Moving down south and below 42nd Street I had the most amazing view of the New York Public Library. The MetLife building behind my desk would reflect the sunsets like an Inca monument, and to my right still, the Empire State building even more grand with age. I did some of my best thinking staring at these urban trophies scattered across town that reached to the sky—unfazed by the activities that were happening below from street corner to street corner.

I returned home and sat at my desk staring out at the George Washington Bridge and the Hudson River and thought, 'what am I going to do now?'

Then it hit me. What if I took my new Avon career to the street- move out of the corner office to the street corner - to talk to women about beauty? I could still use the Avon catalogue and product as an incentive to my interviewees for their time while I created the opportunity to sit with women face to face and talk about what was on their mind when the topic was beauty, product and celebrity. The list that I had created under Genevieve's watchful eye would be my starting point.

The more I thought about hitting the street in search of beauty insights the more excited I became. Having been in the beauty industry for over thirty years I knew the importance of listening to what women were saying. A.G. Laffley, the CEO of Procter and Gamble, was always very clear about the company's mantra, "Consumers are boss". A. G. zeroed in on a fundamental element to successfully market products. Consumer insight is the fuel that runs the communication machine. Decades before, David Ogilvy reminded us early on in the evolution of brand communications that " the consumer is your wife". With beauty brands competing to attract buyers, I believe it would be the one who listens best that would reap the rewards.

In the world of consumer research there are professionals and facilities that provide a great service. Often companies conduct focus groups to understand if a product or advertising concept will appeal to prospective consumers. A negative reaction to an idea could be the end to the creative process. While this is a very simplified illustration of the multimillion-dollar consumer research industry, I have often wondered if probing a bit further with the right questions might lead to other results. My recent experience with this type of situation was rather interesting.

The L'Oreal Paris slogan, "Because You're Worth It", and its relevance, was being questioned. There were camps forming both at the agency and the client that were pro and con for the forty plus year old mantra of "worth". Because of manipulated research results the slogan was almost abandoned. A slogan that is perhaps one of the most recognized beauty statements the world has known was almost dismissed, or replaced, due to an inability to listen to what women were really saying about beauty and the value of worth. I believe the motivation was partly due to a "not invented here" attitude among some of the newer players on both the agency and client side. I also think that situation provided me with an even greater desire to seek out consumer truth.

The enthusiasm that Genevieve ignited was now being fueled by the possibilities that I saw ahead of me in conducting my own research that would explore the things I wanted to better understand from women about beauty. This for me became a unique opportunity to find out how women felt on the topic in the context of today's world.

With this plan in mind I needed to create a "how to" research kit. In the past there would be a strategic planner or consumer research group that would take charge at this point. But as a newly inspired "independent researcher" and Avon sales representative, I was about to do it all. The thing I realized about this independence was that there was less time spent persuading others that what I had in mind was a good idea; rather it allowed more time to get it done. In business I had learned it was best to apologize afterwards than ask for permission up front - a philosophy that served me well. This approach always seemed to yield greater productivity.

Starting with my Pro-Book and a Power Point tool, I began to outline the areas that I was interested in learning more about from women. There was the standard opening query of "tell me about your beauty routine" that would get women into the topic and from there I could become more specific about products, brands, and celebrities. At this point I only had some Avon samples and brochures. I needed to expand this beyond Avon so I decided to visit a local Kmart to buy some additional products. This in itself garnered one of many insights on what a woman deals with trying to decide which product is the right one for her.

In the beauty business we call them "store checks"—the practice of checking on your product and the competition in the store environment. It was something we would do from time to time as a professional group. It was something I did every time I went into a store, no matter where and no matter what. It became a habit even if my sole purpose for being there was to pick up a roll of paper towels. It was a sense of responsibility that I felt was part of my career in beauty. I would stand and rearrange shampoo bottles that had been turned with the labels facing the wrong way or line up the lipstick tubes so that the shade names were easily noticeable. Each time I would take a step back and review the competition that flanked the brand that I was leading, dismissing with a degree of prejudice the messy packaging graphics or the lesser quality plastic containers that they used. This time my 'in-store' mission was different. I was there as a consumer to purchase beauty products and not to "store check" on them.

Standing in the beauty section at Kmart looking at a range of products to my right and left, up and down, I thought to myself, 'with all these choices, how do everyday women shopping for beauty products begin to figure any of this out?' My first stop on the beauty buying express was in the cosmetic section.

Cosmetics are broken into sub-segments that include lip, nail, eye and face. Within each of these segments, a company like L'Oreal or Cover Girl, can have multiple brands and versions. This can lead to an overwhelming supply of choices. Long wear, moisturizing, intense pigment, glossy, creamy, non-feathering (won't seep into the lines around your lips), 24 hour, 48 hour, honey infused, vitamin included, SPF protection, flavored, etc., are examples of what a women standing looking for a red lip stick would have to confront. This mutates into multiple brands that stretch across shelves that can be over thirty feet long. When you step back all you see is an endless sea of posters featuring beautiful celebrities and models with shiny metal, glass or plastic containers filled with a variety of product. That is what one encounters in a store aisle looking for a shade of Passion Pink. Can you imagine what the beauty journey is like moving on to foundations, face powders, concealers, mascara, eyeliners, eye shadows, nail polish, all with a variety of benefits, product forms and, of course, beauty promises?!

It may have seemed odd to the women around me that I was filling my cart with all this stuff. I even noticed that some of the women just observed as I made my choices from the selection of products. Perhaps they thought I was a drag queen or maybe a really great husband or both! The fact is that this was the first phase of my research and what I discovered is that women shopping at mass are confronted with an overwhelming offering of beauty products. Having been in the beauty industry for a number of years and watching more and more products enter the market, I'm aware of the vast amount of product from which to choose. For a consumer making selections, it must be a daunting experience.

Once I made my product selections, I moved on to organizing a plan to learn from women how they view the various brands and what drives their attitudes and purchasing decisions.

To accomplish this I would need answers for several questions:

1. What do you want to learn about women and beauty products?
2. Which brands are the best to learn from?
3. Which segments are the most important?
4. How will packaging influence a woman's choice of products?
5. Is price sensitivity equal among the segments?
6. Do ingredients play a role in the purchase decision?
7. Is there brand loyalty across the beauty segments?
8. Can mass skincare brands compete with department store brands on a better value proposition?
9. How does celebrity influence a woman?
10. How important is a brand's image?

I now had a basic strategic map to guide me in the exploration of women and how they really felt about beauty brands.

With that in mind I began to make my choices. I decided I would focus on brand image, product innovation, packaging, technology and celebrity to use as discussion points in my research. In this way I would be able to gain insights on how women look at these areas when it came to the ever-changing offering of products across the various segments.

I continued on to the shampoo and then skin care sections only to be just as overwhelmed by the number of products, variety of packaging and ingredient versions being offered. Was I being tested, just like any consumer, to see how far I could go in making a choice? I recognized all of the products that I was visually scanning having worked on them at one point or having kept track of their competitive advantages or lack there of. This experience gave me deeper insight into how confusing the choice of beauty products could be. I was even more committed to understanding how women maneuver in the maze of "beauty land".

When my selections were finally made I headed to the check out counter. I smiled as the check out lady scanned and recorded my beauty picks. Since I used my credit card the retailer now had my choices on record – valuable data for both the retailer and beauty companies. The check out lady was entertained by the amount of product that I had chosen. The purchase that afternoon totaled over six hundred dollars. While it was money spent in the pursuit of beauty insights, I realized the stuff isn't cheap. I hoped that the choices I had made would be worth it.

Beautiful You

Once in awhile you stop and have to say to yourself 'what are you doing?' I mean 'what was the point I was trying to get to?' Was I looking for the new silver bullet to selling beauty or was I being honest in my pursuit of a deeper understanding of women and beauty? Or was I using this exercise as a distraction from my unemployment? I wasn't sure but at this point I had tons of products as well as Avon brochures and catalogues lined up on my table. Up until now it was about collecting information, what the digital world refers to as the "discovery phase". Now the challenge was to figure out what to do with it all. It would have been easy to review the information and provide my own point of view on it, but the point was to listen to what women thought about it. It became apparent to me that when I was in the company of other beauty professionals we had a short hand based on collective experience and knowledge. Sometimes we were speaking with authority, basic lessons learned, or sometimes, intelligent but risky speculation. We often tried to out maneuver our competition by obtaining in-store sales materials that might give us a heads up on what they might be up to. It was a game and every beauty company played it. Retail relationships are valuable.

We did from time to time ask women what they thought but more often it was after our plans were made to confirm that our instinctual expertise was correct. We often would take a wait and see approach if we didn't hear what we wanted hoping that the idea would eventually catch on. When it did we were proven right and when it didn't we would often try to fix it. Most of the time the fixes were too late, as once the marketing plan was sold to a big retailer like a Walmart there was no turning back. I often felt that if we had talked and more importantly listened to women up front, we may have avoided some of our failed product launches. This is what happens with decision by committee! While we operated in a culture where our collective enthusiasm for success outweighed the possibility of failure, in the end, everyday women would be the judge and have the final say.

I kept looking at the products on the table and thought that I had this incredible one-on-one opportunity to understand what women really thought about all of this stuff. In front of me was a collection of beauty products that actually made it to market. Getting it there is an expensive process.

A new product launch can take years of research and development, testing formulas for efficacy and product stability and, as all beauty manufactures well know, the competition may be on your heels and "time is money". The process begins with what's called Concept Development to determine the product interest among potential consumers. There can often be up to ten different concepts tested with slight variations on what the product does or how it might be positioned to consumers. Once consumers indicate which concept or concepts they prefer, the refinements for communication begins. The variants here could be overwhelming, from typeface to packaging and product descriptors in multiples. To determine the best ones to capture consumer interest or what in the business is called "purchase intent" can take months to complete. The communication tool for a brand's new product launch can be in the form of digital or traditional that includes print and TV or, in today's multichannel world, all three. Once the creative execution is developed it is be tested to determine its effectiveness in building brand or product awareness and the interest to try or purchase it. If the product formula or benefit was not more effective than the competition, or breakthrough in the category then the challenge of creating the impression that it was became the responsibility of the brand communications across public relations, advertising, digital and social media.

All along the way adjustments and refinements are made to correct any issues that would surface. For example, product stability or testing for superiority claims versus the competition. If a new product didn't meet the criteria for launch it might be filed away for another time when its benefit became something a person might really want or at least consider.

The question that would come to mind each time is how is it "better" and "different"? More importantly, I think the consideration should have also included 'does anyone need it?' Of course this is a very broad and perhaps simplistic explanation of an industry's approach to compete in the beauty world. But, in its simplicity, it would always harken back to a fundamental flaw that can be addressed through simple dialogue. Unilever attempted this back in 2002 with a global research project that set out to discover what women really wanted from beauty.

"The Real Truth About Beauty" was the name of the Unilever project for Dove. The outcome of this research was "The Dove Campaign for Real Beauty" which premiered in 2004. For those of us in the beauty business it was a disruption in the category of how a company talks about beauty to women. I remember walking through an airport in Japan looking up at enormous banners that advertised its arrival. Like others in my field I sat back and waited to see what impact it would have on beauty. On a personal level it made me aware that in order for brands to remain relevant and connected there was a need for change in they way beauty companies talked to women.

The global research conducted in ten countries included thirty-two hundred women over a period of two months. To me the most staggering finding in the study was this: of the women contacted only two percent described themselves as beautiful. Can you image that of the thirty-two hundred women in the study only sixty-four considered themselves beautiful? I believe that the study revealed to Unilever that a reframing of what it means to feel beautiful would be a historic breakthrough in the industry. In their attempt they were noticed and celebrated for the honesty they communicated in their advertising to women. Perhaps in their internal dialogue they missed an important insight on women. In my opinion, while the majority of women may not feel they are beautiful, every woman still has the desire to be just that. It is a fine line that separates the two ideas but I have never met a woman who doesn't want to try to be her best and to expect more out of life. The beauty category can only be "beautiful" if it has an element of intrigue, delight and magic. It became my mission to understand the value of feeling beautiful and how the offerings at Kmart, Walmart, even Saks, or wherever they shopped, can help to make a woman feel that way.

It was now time to develop an approach to my research based on the three elements that I had at hand. First my Avon Kit, second the products purchased at Kmart and third, an idea to discover the relevance of beauty today among women.

In my approach to discover the real meaning of beauty among women I purposely did not include any form of advertising. The reason for that was I didn't want the conversation with women to turn into a critique on print or television creative executions. In my career I had become well aware that women judging other women in ads could veil the true feeling they had about beauty care and, after all, Dove had done that given their Real Beauty campaign and the critique of the beauty industry that resulted.

So where do you begin talking to women about beauty? Each of the interviews would start with a broader probe on the topic by asking them to just talk about beauty care. In every interview the women would pause to consider what that question meant. It ranged from a functional need to an aspirational desire, all of which provided a more insightful dialogue that was about them and how they felt about beauty care.

The Women

I t has been documented that the phrase "Beauty is in the eye of the beholder" was first spoken in the third century BC in Greece. Its literal meaning is that the idea of beauty is subjective. With that in mind it was important to have the right tools and questions to help bring some order to this subjective topic.

I knew that if the interviewees were friends of mine the conversations would be different so I asked my female friends if they would introduce me to their female friends. Then I was able to ask the first dozen interviewees if they would introduce me to some of their friends and before I knew it the "sample", as we call it in the business, began to mushroom. With this approach I was able to conduct one-on-one interviews and get to the honest insights I was seeking. The kitsch factor of being an Avon representative was on my mind as well so I was clear up front that the Avon element was only a part of what I was hoping to explore with them. I needed a balanced approach to understand how women really felt about beauty.

The women were a cross section of professionals and stay at home moms. They were from both urban and rural areas. They were cooks and business executives, interns and secretaries from all walks of life with different life experience. They shopped at Sephora in NYC, and a Walmart in PA; they had disposable income and household budgets to work within. Many were college educated some were not; they were moms, daughters, sisters and wives who were willing to talk about the relevance of beauty today in their own words. In the end their collective feelings, aspirations and desires were universal and they mainly pursued beauty for themselves, to make them not only look better but feel better.

I started with a few women in rural areas (close to my country house), where access to product was mainly in the large chain outlets that exist across America. Retailers in the area that I am referring to included Walmart, Kmart, CVS and locally owned family grocery stores. This group represented about half of all the women in the sample of women that I interviewed. The women in the rural environment were not all mass brand users. A few of them had relocated from urban cities and remained brand loyal to department store brands. The women who were born in this country setting were also the most knowledgeable about Avon and Mary Kay. A few had a relative or friend that was a sale representative for either one. Affordability was a larger concern among all age levels in this group. Only those that relocated from various cities talked about the "good old days" when they could run into a department store and pick up their favorite skin care or cosmetic product. When questioned, none of the women in this group shopped for beauty products on the Internet or QVC/HSN. They were extremely loyal to brands once they found something that worked, and, although they would be influenced by new products that reflected the latest trend, they were often more concerned about how it would impact their budget. In their words any product in skin care nearing the price point of twenty dollars "better work".

The other fifty percent of women interviewed were from urban areas. This group was split between twenty to thirty year old women and those that were forty plus. The youngest in this group was twenty the oldest was over sixty-five years old. While these women shared an urban lifestyle, they were the most diverse when it came to ethnicity, income and education.

The majority worked in professional environments, while a few were no longer employed. The difference in demographics among this group did not directly correlate to mass or prestige users. Among this group there was a greater awareness of new products and trends in fashion. They were the most diverse group when it came to shopping the various classes of trade, drug, department and mass stores. When they were in search of product information the majority relied on department store sales professionals or destinations like Sephora and MAC to learn more. Even though they obtained product information in these places it did not always covert into a sale. With the in-store learning the younger group would look for alternative products in mass at a lower price containing the same ingredient or offering a similar benefit.

Both age groups did look to the Internet for education on products and, in general, they were label readers when it came to skin care. Advertising was not a big source of information for them mostly due to the skepticism they felt with the way women were overly retouched, or made up by professional stylists and makeup artists for the commercials and print ads. Similar to the rural group of women, urban women were concerned about cost but were willing to pay more for better quality products. In this case they would create a pecking order of importance whereby they would spend a bit more for one product and less on another. Here the pecking order was not universal, rather it depended on what beauty segment they felt was more important to them.

Overall the interviewees were very willing to talk about beauty care. Some embraced it as an opportunity to express themselves. In every interview they were delighted with the experience to just talk beauty and found it refreshing that there was someone interested in what they had to say.

The interviews maintained an element of consistency however they were fluid enough to allow room for dialogue to go off on tangents. In those cases if I hit upon a new insight on beauty I would incorporate it into the next interview. The end result of all the interviews provided a greater understanding of the importance that beauty products still have in women's lives. Furthermore, importance of beauty care among the women in the interviews was far more individualistic than the broader beliefs that the beauty industry maintains.

Let's Talk

did not interview thirty-two hundred women for this informal but focused study. In fact I only interviewed one hundred. After the first dozen the consistency among women on beauty became obvious, but I went on to interview a few dozen more. Along the way universal insights emerged quickly. Individual expressions of beauty did as well, making the intimacy of this study more valuable to both the woman and myself. I learned quickly to allow the women I spoke with to do more of the talking. This is a lesson I learned long ago, be a good listener. Let them tell you how they feel and don't put words in their mouth or lead them in the exchange. Earlier I mentioned the shorthand that develops with people in a shared career; well, here it would not apply because it would only yield what we in the corner offices already knew, or thought we did, about women and beauty.

My first interview was in early May. I prepared the setting with product that remained in a camouflaged Cookie Magazine nylon tote (from a wonderful publication no longer on the stands). Inside were plastic Ziploc bags that contained various products from five major cosmetic companies, two skin care lines and a variety of shampoos.

I told the women what I wanted to talk about with them, asked if I could record the conversation, and then I handed them an Avon catalogue. In the beginning of the series of interviews I asked them to select ten products from the catalogue. Once the interview was complete I would ask them if they wanted to change any of their choices. The objective here was to understand if based on the conversation they would switch products. (This approach needed to be revised given the time it took to review all the choices in the Avon catalogue. The diversity of products went beyond beauty, which became an obstacle). This early learning became a focal point when discussing the Avon brand, which is detailed later on in this study. What I ultimately did was to ask them to select 5 products which I would then purchase and send to them as a follow up thank you for their participation. This was also an important element to keep my Avon account status active. I believe in addition to the initial investment made on the purchase of the various beauty products, a further investment of over five hundred dollars was made on the purchasing of Avon product. Sadly, it was not nearly enough to qualify for the trip to Alaska…

I would begin the interview with the same words that Genevieve used only weeks earlier when I met her at Avon's East Harlem Headquarters, "Let's talk".

'How do you approach beauty care?' was the first question I asked each of the interviewees. The first thing I observed after asking the question is how each of the interviewees reacted to the question. The majority would smile then begin talking about beauty routines or products. There were also those interviewees that took a moment to think about the topic and then begin to talk about their individual needs. The universal commonality among the interviewees is that they approached the topic with great thoughtfulness. This was the first validation of my belief that beauty continues to be both relevant and personal for women.

Within the first dozen women interviewed a pattern emerged on how they approached the topic of beauty. There were four points of entry on the topic that quickly emerged with all the interviews: skin, cosmetics, hair and, finally 'no interest' (stay tuned). Listed here are these four points of entry on the topic and summarized in the order of most important to the least mentioned.

1. The majority of interviewees with whom I spoke talked about the importance of their skin care. Skincare or "clean and beautiful skin" is what defined beauty in their life with healthy skin as the foundation of their beauty. The women in this group described their daily routine and mentioned a variety of products and rituals for day and night. This group firmly believed that cleansing and moisturizing were the basis for beauty. This notion had been reinforced, as many suggested, by advice received by Mother.

The majority of interviewees believed that healthy skin was the starting point to beauty. From adolescent memories of acne, to concerns over lines and wrinkles, women considered taking care of their skin as the number one priority. In speaking to the older women, while they shared the same concern over sun damage, it was obvious that younger women were far more aware of the negative effects of the sun on the skin. Many mentioned that they relied on the Internet to learn more about sun damage prevention. It was this younger interviewee that would seek out and use products, beyond skin care, containing SPF protection. Many of the women interviewed avoided tanning outdoors using available bronzing products instead to capture a healthy glow.

The range of products covered three areas; cleansers, moisturizers, and anti-aging creams. Mostly they aligned with the various ages and needs. Interestingly some of the younger women mentioned that they were using anti-aging products for early prevention against lines and wrinkles.

Maintaining healthy looking skin was the entry point for the majority of the interviewees and it went beyond the topic of skin care products and cleaners. This group, besides being concerned about sun damage, were also much more in-touch about the need for a healthy diet, exercise, and sleep to maintain that "healthy glow" of their skin.

This group of interviewees believed that healthy skin was the foundation of their beauty. They were a cross section of all ages (twenty to sixty-plus), ethnicities, and incomes. Their geographic location (city or country) did not influence their feelings about the relationship between healthy skin and a healthy lifestyle.

2. The second most popular entry point on the topic of beauty care focused on cosmetic products. What distinguished this group of

interviewees from those that talked about skin care was their passion for color and cosmetics as tools for self-expression. This was surprisingly consistent across all the women interviewed. The women using this entry point to discuss beauty seemed far more animated when they described what they liked about cosmetics.

For this group, their experience with cosmetics had strong association with mothers and girlfriends who were the greatest influencers in this segment but for different reason. Mothers, for the basics, and mostly stemming from childhood "dress up" and using moms make up. Early lessons learned on application was key here—"watching mom apply lip color and mascara". Girlfriends mentioned by most of the interviewees had a great deal of influence on helping them to experiment with different make up looks. A small percentage of this segment were active on the Internet learning about application and the "how to" approach to getting a specific look. The younger women talked about cosmetics mentioned beauty video bloggers like Michelle Phan and her posts on YouTube as a source for inspiration and information.

Most women have a cosmetic routine that is based on season, day or night, and special occasions where the degree of product used varies. Seasonality influences color choices, pastels in spring and summer, nudes and darker shade for winter and fall. What is true about this group is the desire to "play" more with color, but it is not a regular routine. Many interviewees mentioned that when they look back on the special occasions in their life they wished they did not go to the extreme to cover up who they are with makeup that marked the occasion because it did not reflect the real person under it all. Often they compared this feeling with fad fashion choices and crazy hairstyles that were a sign of the times. We have all looked back at prom or wedding photos and thought, "what was I thinking?"

Eye products, like mascara, liners, shadows and pencils were the predominant make up tools they used. The idea that eyes can be enhanced without looking too overdone was common and was incorporated into their daily routine. Color was mainly for evening and winter months because "evening lighting" was an important factor in enhancing a look and winter because color helped to lift ones spirit from the "grey" season.

Foundations were important during winter for protection and not that desirable during warmer weather. The biggest concern about foundations was the "fake" or "overly made up look" that was associated with the products. Skin tone mismatching and streaking effects were negatives that could be overcome with the help of department sales staff. Many of the interviewees mentioned this is how they would find the best match for their skin tone, and then try to find the equivalent product at mass. Women who were loyal to department store foundations were very clear that they would never "try" or "use" a mass brand.

Lip color and nail color are staples for every woman in the group. The women became very animated talking about their preference; "rich and bright colors for evening" and "nudes, flesh tones and glosses for day time". All the women in this segment mentioned specific brands, both prestige and mass when it came to nail, lip and mascara. In this area of color cosmetics there was far less resistance among the interviewees in terms of crossing over between mass and department store brands.

The interviewees who entered the topic on beauty using cosmetics as the point of entry were as diverse as the women who talked about their skin. I found it interesting that the two groups would never be identified by physical characteristics. In other words, the women who talked about healthy skin looked no different from the women who began the conversation talking about cosmetics. The difference, however, was more psychographic which is how they talked and felt about it. Unlike the interviewees who were rather serious and responsible in their approach to beauty and healthy skin, the second group who talked first about cosmetics was far more spirited when it came to the topic, as it was more about the "look" and less about "care".

3. The third entry point on beauty care was the interviewee that talked about their hair and hair care products. This group was bonded by an endless pursuit to find the right product for them. Their focus was very problem/solution oriented. As passionate as the first two groups, the women who started the conversation talking about hair care talked about "her beauty" from the perspective of their own hair. For me it was a shared passion given my personal experience on the subject. Hair care many years ago was also my first entry into beauty. In 1986 I was hired to work at a boutique-advertising agency. Peter Rogers Associates was the agency for Vidal

Sassoon, the legendary stylist from the 60's. It was Peter that created the infamous slogan *"If you don't look good, we don't look good"*.

On the topic of hair care, and despite the proliferation in the category of multiple product lines and benefits, these interviewees were constantly searching for the answer to their hair issues and problems. Hair care was the backbone to their beauty and this group was almost obsessive about the importance of a "good hair day".

Interviewees were somewhat realistic about what was achievable based on what type of hair they had, however they were constantly trying new products in the hope they could have thicker, fuller, smoother, stronger, shinier, longer, manageable, softer hair.

In this group shampooing was the start to the day and thus associated with beauty. Shampooing seemed, in the context of beauty, to be more functional then anything else. Some associated the water, lather, and scent as a catalyst to wake them up in the morning. While functional, women did describe this as more problem solution in the attempt to achieve volume or control frizz.

Scent and texture were predominating beauty elements when they talked about their morning routine. Brand switching is a known fact in this segment that the interviewees confirmed. The switching simply takes place because women believe over time a favored brand "stops working". Neutrogena, back in the late eighties, created an entire business with one of their shampoos by simply leveraging this consumer belief. They advertised that if you felt that your current shampoo was no longer effective then, "switch for 14 days" to theirs. This belief among women still exists that any shampoo after a certain amount of time losses its effectiveness requiring one to switch off to a different one.

Because of the constant search for the perfect shampoo, women tend to not be brand loyal in this segment. If there was any loyalty it was towards salon brands that were recommended to them by a stylist. Word of mouth or consumer reviews, mainly in social media, provides greater influence on what women in this group said they would try.

4. The fourth entry point on the topic of beauty care among women interviewed, were the interviewees that stated they were not that interested in beauty care. This group of women claimed that they were "minimalists" when it came to using beauty products.

These interviewees were clearly in the minority. Among all the women, she was the woman who talked about a lack of beauty interest and said she used very few products. Some of the interviewees took great pride almost to a point of defiance that they were not interested in beauty products other than gentle soap and some moisturizer for their skin.

Interestingly for me their appearance did not totally reflect their attitude about beauty product usage. These interviewees were made up mainly of urban professionals. Their appearance would lead you to believe they were definitely beauty product involved. In dissecting the conversation further I began to think it was more perception on their part then anything else.

What they did and how they defined "use" was more about minimal coverage and products, but not complete abstinence from products. A simple mascara and lip balm was enough for daytime at the office; in the evening they added a bit of lip color and eye shadow. Nail color was used, but mostly nude and pale pink tones applied here. For this group of interviewees it was obvious to me that they used a fair amount of product and did not necessarily "practice what they preached". Claiming to be minimalist they were still using products to "enhance" their features.

The interviewees in this last entry point on the topic of beauty were often the youngest among all the women interviewed. It was clear that their statements were more about not being defined by beauty. However when they talked about what "minimal" product they used, to my surprise, it was nearly as much product as the women who started the conversation on beauty talking about cosmetics!

Another interesting insight learned from this cluster of inter-viewees or "minimalists", is that while they considered themselves less interested in beauty, in fact, they were the most informed. As beauty product minimalists they were the most critical of harsh ingredients and animal testing. Among all the groups this one clearly expressed a desire for more natural products and "green" packaging. This group spent a great deal of time researching products on-line which seemed to contradict their low interest on the topic of beauty products. Given their "fact gathering interest" on beauty products, they were also the group that were mixing and creating their own beauty elixirs including scrubs, face and eye creams and facial mists. The irony here was while they proclaimed to have little interest in beauty care at the onset of the conversation they proved to be far more educated on products.

From this first exercise some interesting insights emerged.

Women do not approach the topic of beauty in the same manner. They simply viewed the topic of beauty care in relationship to their daily lives and early influences. This learning only underscored how subjective and vast the topic of beauty is and that what may be the beginning of a conversation for one on the topic may have very little interest for another. It was far more practical than I expected.

Interviewees who were influenced from childhood that "healthy skin" is the foundation of beauty learned this mostly from their mothers. This was in their minds the basis of beauty from which all other products and regimes would follow. Beauty for this woman was the result of a healthy glow from good skin rather than the application of layers of products.

When interviewees talked about cosmetics being the focal point on beauty they expressed their delight in experimenting and finding what worked best for them. These women took pleasure in the application of make up and spoke with a degree of confidence on which facial feature needed more or less enhancement through the use of product.

The interviewee that began with their hair and hair care needs saw this as the center of their beauty. For this woman she was mainly looking for a product that would work to improve her hair. Her beauty seemed more functional and problem/solution oriented. Other than mentioning the importance of scent and packaging it seemed her frame of reference on the topic of beauty was relegated to the morning shower. For this group finding the "right product" was key to having beautiful hair, which defined beauty for them.

The women, mostly younger, interviewed that stated beauty products were the least important thing to them seemed to be somewhat of a contradiction as it was clear that they all used cosmetics. The most interesting insight discovered by interviewing women who saw themselves as not all that involved in beauty practices is that she seemed to be the best informed when it came to product and ingredients.

When talking about beauty care on a personal level, women felt comfortable addressing the topic based on what they did in their daily routines, what had influenced them and, most importantly, how comfortable they felt about their own beauty. The underlying insight was the importance that was placed on care and overall beauty enhancement. Not one interviewee ever mentioned how she wished she looked different. When one did mention a desire for smoother hair or healthier skin it was in the context of what they do to achieve it in a proactive way.

Lastly, I found it interesting that celebrities were never mentioned, nor were industry catch phrases like "radiant skin", "silky, shiny hair" or "revolutionary wrinkle repair". The language was very straight forward, practical, and simple when talking to the interviewees about what beauty care meant to them.

Sassy or Sophisticated

With an understanding of what beauty care meant to the women interviewed, next in the plan was to understand what brand images were conjured up in minds of interviewees at the mention of a beauty brand's name. The competitive set used to probe the topic of brand image included Maybelline, Cover Girl, L'Oreal Paris, Revlon and Avon, each with a rich and interesting history.

Without the use of advertising or product packaging, the women were asked 'what comes to mind, or what is your first impression of the following brands?' The brands selected back at Kmart were all mass cosmetic brands. The five cosmetic brands selected were all global brands and have been in existence for decades so I expected that the women interviewed would have a frame of reference for each. It turned out that every interviewee was familiar with the competitive set of brands selected and they all had strong impressions of what each one represented.

For background (and some fun) here are a few details about each brand.

Maybelline is known for it's superior market share in cosmetics with their mascara called Great Lash. It's not surprising why. The company was founded in 1914 by a chemist named T.L. Williams. As the story goes, the idea for mascara for this company started because Mr. Williams observed his little sister applying a small amount of Vaseline mixed with coal dust to her eyelashes. He called it "Lash-Brow-Lne" and while women liked the results the name was never a hit. His sister, Mabel, was not only the inspiration for the product, but also the product name, Maybelline. The brand slogan "Maybe she's born with it. Maybe it's Maybelline", created in 1991, continues on today.

Next we have **Cover Girl**. In 1960 Noxzema Chemical Company launched the brand known today as Cover Girl. The name is synonymous with the practice of featuring models on the cover of fashion and beauty magazines. The first face for this cosmetic brand was Jennifer O'Neill who was a model until her film debut in the movie "The Summer of 42" premiered in 1971. The then model turned actress was a Cover Girl for over thirty years and led the company to success. Another model turned actress who was the face of the brand was Cybil Shepherd. Ironically Cybil was also the face of L'Oreal's Preference Hair Color for a number of years following her relationship with Cover Girl. Known for its "girl next door" tonality, Christie Brinkley continued the model tradition format of the brand with a relationship with the brand that lasted twenty-five years.

A chemist by the name Eugene Schueller founded **L'Oreal** in 1907. This Frenchman created the first hair dye which he sold to hair stylists in Paris. The product was called "Aureale", which translated into English means "crowned glory or halo". This singular product would mark the beginning of what has become the largest beauty company today. Given Mr. Schueller's passion for science and discovery, the company's guiding principles, then and now, are rooted in research and innovation. Today, a known fact about L'Oreal is that the company holds more patents and employs more scientists than any other global beauty product company. Their investment in research and development is at the core of their existence. L'Oreal is a company comprised of multiple brands including Lancome, Redkin, Maybelline, Urban Decay and Garnier, just to mention a few. The company's infamous slogan for its mass brand L'Oreal Paris, "Because I'm Worth it", was created by a young copywriter in 1973.

Her name is Ilon Specht and as the story goes, she was working with a group of 'Mad Men' account types at McCann Erickson on the launch of a new hair color, Superior Preference. It was L'Oreal Paris (the brand) first major U.S. product launch. At the time Clairol's Nice n Easy held the majority share of the at home hair color market. L'Oreal Paris had invested heavily in developing a superior hair color but unfortunately neglected to invest in consumer trials that would allow the company to make superiority claims versus its competitor Clairol's "Nice 'n Easy".

With a launch date looming, it was the twenty-three year-old Ms. Specht who saved the day not to mention created one of the most well known slogans in advertising history. A little know fact about this slogan is that while it was introduced in 1973, it was only used in the Superior Preference Hair Color communications in the U.S. In 1997 Lindsey Owens Jones, a Welshman and the CEO at that time, mandated that it become the corner stone mantra for L'Oreal Paris worldwide-much to the chagrin of the French (after all it was an American invention)! I was there in Paris for the world-wide summit, and proudly created, with a few colleagues at McCann Erickson in New York, the "Purple Book" which documented the L'Oreal mission statement and the renewed commitment to women and empowerment to mark the occasion.

The fourth brand to be studied is **Revlon**. Charles and Joseph Revson founded this iconic American brand in 1931. The brothers teamed up with chemist Charles Lachman to develop a new form of nail enamel based on pigments and not dyes. By the 1940's they added lipstick and soon Revlon became a successful multimillion-dollar cosmetic company. In addition to its innovation at the very start, Revlon was also the first to expand in terms of diversity and to feature an African American woman in advertising. In 1992 Veronica Webb represented a line of products targeted to women of color. Revlon was one of the first American cosmetics brands to go global in the late fifties and by the early sixties had distribution in Europe, Latin America and Asia. When launching the brand in Japan the company decided to use the American advertising. That proved to be a smart strategy as the women of Japan loved the American look and the brand took off resulting in strong sales.

The final brand in the mix is **Avon**. In the beginning of the book I write a lot about the origin of this American brand. In the brand's long heritage, it has expanded beyond beauty and into household, fashion accessories and personal care products. Avon is sold in more than one hundred and forty countries globally and is represented by over six million sales representatives around the world. The fifties and sixties advertising campaign, "Ding Dong, Avon Calling" remains to this day strongly associated with the brand-something that may be to the brand's disadvantage.

With a snapshot of the five brands in the probe on image we now move on to the unaided responses among the women on brand impression.

Maybelline is described by most of the women interviewed as a lower end or a starter brand. Youth is strongly associated with this brand. This is primarily driven by the brand's color code and packaging. It does have a number of positives, one of which was the mascara's longevity, superior performance and product reliability.

Most of the older interviewees referenced the brand as the one they used when they were still in school and couldn't afford better. It was also described as a brand that you can pick up "if you are in a pinch because you left your favorite mascara at home". In the minds of the women the bold hot pink and vivid green are still color codes closely associated with the Maybelline brand.

Recently the brand has been making great efforts to drive a more sophisticated image both in the advertising and in packaging. This new look was just being seeded at the time of these interviews with a new foundation called "Fit Me". The task of evolving a brand image and the impressions women may have can take some time, especially a brand with a very clear and distinct image like Maybelline.

Maybelline is the one brand that has made quite the effort to evolve the brand image to a more sophisticated place. Brand communications and upgraded packaging is working to evolve this brand from its "cheap" image to one of greater value. This evolution would mostly impact and attract younger users to the brand. For the women that I interviewed this evolution wouldn't be as noticeable since their strong impression of the brand would not be easily changed regardless of the brand's new look.

Cover Girl is on the opposite end of the spectrum from Maybelline in the minds of the interviewees. If Maybelline is New York 'urban vamp', then Cover Girl is 'sugar and spice and all things nice'. Women saw Cover Girl as a starter brand, too, and for younger women going off to college. Its longevity in the market has provided some credibility but also has older women remembering Cheryl Teigs as one of the earlier Cover Girls.

The main take away about the brand is that it has a lower price point coupled with lots of celebrities. When probed which celebrities were representing the brand most of the interviewees could only recall Queen Latifah and Drew Barrymore (both are no longer spokeswomen for the brand). What I found interesting about the portfolio of women that are spokespeople for the brand is the diversity. From Ellen DeGeneres to Sofia Vergara, Rihanna and Taylor Swift, the brand reflects the diversity of America.

Additional equity associations included Top Model and one reference to the *Easy Breezy* brand tag line. In comparison to Maybelline, the interviewees see Cover Girl as a more natural, less of a flashy brand. None of the women interviewed were using the Cover Girl brand nor would they consider it if they were in need of a lipstick or mascara. The same was not true among some of the interviewees when it came down to using mascara from Maybelline.

L'Oreal Paris was the third to be discussed and the brand that I know best about. I had been part of its brand evolution from the early nineties up until this project and therefore particularly interested in understanding from the group their impressions of the brand.

The women interviewed believe L'Oreal Paris to be a very good product. It was considered to be a step above both Maybelline and Cover Girl. References for the company range from nice colors to shampoo, hair color, and "no nonsense performance". Women separate this brand from others in mass referring to it as an "adult" brand and more upscale. The interviewees in the group were far more animated when they described the brand image of L'Oreal Paris versus Maybelline and Cover Girl. Even if the interviewees were not L'Oreal Paris users they were able to relate to the strong brand image. Words used to describe it included, "elegant", "French chic", "celebrity" and "red carpet".

Women view the brand as a higher quality product, however that association also meant to the interviewees a more "expensive brand". They felt that the price point, even though it was more, was worth it. As one woman said, "It speaks for itself". L'Oreal's longevity, like Cover Girl, has both a positive and negative effect. The women interviewed remember it as a brand "my mother used", or because it was around for a period of time, it was considered to be "tried and true". As one of the interviewees put it, "It's the best of the products, the one I would buy. I used the waterproof mascara on my wedding day."

Women recall that the brand has a lot of celebrities, but most of them could only recall one successfully and that was Andie MacDowell. It was interesting that women would suggest names that they thought were part of the portfolio but the majority had a difficult time, like with Cover Girl, recalling who were the spokes-women for the brand.

In general the interviewees thought that there was a consistent style about the L'Oreal Paris brand. It was a brand that had a clear image of sophistication and quality. While seen as the more expensive brand at mass, it was also seen as the better choice brand and, in some cases, it was because women knew about Lancôme, a department store brand owned by the same company. They expected it was the same product in less expensive packaging.

The L'Oreal Paris slogan "Because I'm Worth It", was referenced by all of interviewees I talked to. It was still viewed as relevant and meaningful to most of them. Similar to Maybelline's "Maybe she's born with It." The L'Oreal Paris slogan is closely associated with the brand. The statement of "worth" and the L'Oreal Paris name are inextricable. Women responded by referencing both the empowerment factor of the slogan communicated as well as a reference to product quality. However, there were those interviewees, mostly the younger women, who felt that a message of empowerment meant very little coming from a company such as L'Oreal, or any product company.

Revlon has the oldest impression according to the women interviewed. Women referenced it as a brand "my mother used" but not in the same positive way they referenced L'Oreal Paris. In this case the association among the interviewed women was old fashioned and dated. In the group of brands discussed so far it had greater credibility over Cover Girl, but was seen as a less expensive, lower end brand in line with Maybelline and was often referred to as a "cheap brand".

Lip color and nail polish are quickly associated with Revlon, which is not surprising, given its heritage. Red is the predominant color in the interviewees' minds when they think of the brand. Revlon has an association with celebrity but the celebrities could not be identified. When the interviewees referenced a celebrity association they were always incorrect with mentions of Julia Roberts and Nikki Taylor.

The women in my study considered Revlon an older brand with cheap nail polish and packaging referenced as "Donald Trump black and gold". It was nowhere close to their impression of L'Oreal Paris. Women continued to mention the nail polish was good but that everything else to them was pretty much a blurring of images that all blended together with Maybelline and Cover Girl.

Revlon's low end, one note "red" image in the minds of the women interviewed limited the discussion about the brand. The brand has been in the process of a make over starting a couple of years ago. The brand has begun a brand renovation with new products, packaging and personalities, the likes of Emma Stone, to appeal to younger women. Following these interviews I have seen a great deal of the new Revlon advertising. Moving away from using black and gold (which now it seems L'Oreal Paris is using) and showcasing celebrities in real settings and daylight is helping to modernize this brand. The new pastel brand codes are evolving Revlon's look to a more feminine and playful place. Emma Stone embodies this new brand sensibility as well. Looking into the future I would predict that this re-imaging of the brand will begin to attract a younger woman given the brand's fresh approach to both it product and communications. However, more recent advertising for the brand has introduced an element of male appreciation (girl gets noticed by guy), and a new slogan "Love is on" which feels oddly less fresh and modern than the former creative.

Avon is synonymous with "Ding Dong, Avon Calling", which plays back with great consistency among women interviewed. In fact, women 40+ remembered the Avon Lady and are well aware of the catalogue of products. However, even with the equity of the Avon Lady and catalogues, there wasn't a clear cut image of this company nor was there any recall of celebrities as part of the brand portfolio.

The brand was described as "antiquated", "old lady", and "women who just sit around". There was some recall of the brand's association with women and breast cancer awareness, but for the most part, the strongest association women had with this brand was door to door Tupperware parties.

"My mom used it", and "the products are pretty cheap", were the most mentioned comments in relation to this brand. There were some interviewees that still shopped the catalogue because they knew someone that was an Avon Representative. The most common product either referenced or purchased was *Skin So Soft* because of its effective use as a mosquito deterrent.

According to the interviewees this study, Avon is the brand that most lacked image, credibility and quality among the majority of interviewees. In fact, the women in the study felt rather neutral about it, or to be blunt, indifferent towards it. One woman commented, "I think it missed a few generations. I think it has become so lost."

The pride Genevieve exuded during my orientation meeting in her East Harlem office was not translating into anything positive or memorable among the women that I spoke to. Was the brand's success in areas of the country where there was little access to beauty products as suggested by one of the interviewees? Or perhaps, suggested by another interviewee, Avon might still appeal to women who are not using the Internet to purchase and still would rely on ordering from a catalogue. All along I wondered why the company did not leverage its heritage of door-to-door service and extensive product line in interactive media, with the potential of becoming the 'Amazon of beauty'. This equity of service in the new digital age of personalization could appeal to a new and younger target.

Avon has never relied on the traditional channels of distribution that include mass, food and drugstores. Instead its long-time advantage selling direct to women would make sense in the emerging area of e-commerce. Like Amazon, the leader in direct selling, Avon could cultivate its loyal user database, either from the one-to-one sales service or the catalogue sales database. Utilizing either, Avon could create a personalized approach to each customer and provide recommendation for products that would be part of the Avon services. Given the diversity of the Avon product categories the possibility of suggestion—a pretty lip gloss to go along with the bejeweled hair clip the customer just ordered—could expand the purchasing by one more product added to the online "shopping cart". In my opinion Avon is prime for a re-invention in both its image and approach cultivating new groups of women while serving their current customer.

As I mentioned earlier, the impressions of all five brands were unaided, that is, without showing any products or visual material like advertising. The interviewee's impressions of each of the five brands were derived from either personal experience or memory. Two insights emerge on the topic of brand impression.

The first is that a brand impression, without advertising or product to evaluate, can live in a women's mind based on a particular time, place and experience. Her familiarity with the brand impression can be locked in a time warp of sorts. Maybelline is a good example of this. If her contact with the brand was during her high school years then that seems to be what her impression of the brand is 30 years later. Unless she is a current user of the brand mentioned it is not part of her mindscape, thus talking about its value is not that easy for her. She relies on what she remembers about the brand, and in most cases the brand has not evolved in her mind. Regardless of a brand's evolution, if it is not part of her routine the image of the brand has little relevance in her life. A brand's relevance to a consumer is essential in driving its value. When the brand name conjures up an old image, regardless of its evolution, it will remain stagnant in her mind. This is further complicated by the vast number of brands that are in the market competing for the attention of the same woman. To her they all begin to look alike.

The second interesting thing learned during this section of the interviews was how little celebrity was mentioned in association with brands. The majority of women were focused on the impression they had of the brand primarily based on their experience with that brand. This is not to say that celebrity was not part of some of the interviews but, in most cases, women struggled to remember which celebrity represented which brands. The only consistency in the brand and celebrity association was Andie MacDowell for L'Oreal Paris and Queen Latifah for Cover Girl.

I find this area of celebrity association to be telling given the amount of effort and expense that goes into selecting a celebrity to represent a brand. Within the five brands in this exercise of brand image, four have a large portfolio of celebrities representing each. The lack of immediate recall, with the exception of a few women referring to recently seeing Jennifer Lopez or Ellen Degeneres in a commercial on television talking about a particular product, is significant. This brand/celebrity connection prompted me to go further in the exploration, which is detailed later on in the study.

With the millions of dollars spent annually on brand building advertising it is interesting that among the women interviewed, advertising was never their point of reference for a brand's image. It is not to say that advertising was not responsible for their overall impressions, rather among the women interviewed it was not top of mind except for an occasional mention of something they had seen recently in a magazine or on TV. The impression of each of the brands was predicated on their personal usage or on a time in the past when they had noticed it. Those images from the past may be where the brand remains in their minds given it has little relevance for them today. For many of the women interviewed the image of the brands discussed was based on where and how the brand fit into their lives. This "fit" included cost, age and any prior product experience.

Product Innovation

n the beauty world of "new, now improved, and never before", unaided brand impressions of the five companies became more specific when "actual product" was introduced into the conversation. The interviewees were able to express how they felt about the packaging, labels, ingredients, and product benefits.

Reaching into my now vintage Cookie Magazine tote I pulled out a sample of various cosmetic products kept in five Ziploc bags. Inside each of the bags was a selection of products representing the same beauty companies previously discussed. I used a black Sharpie pen to indicated the following companies; Maybelline, Cover Girl, L'Oreal Paris, Revlon and Avon. With products in hand the interviewees were far more specific and engaged with each of the brands and the benefit that the product offered them.

The selection of brand products wasn't random. They were selected based on innovation whether it stemmed from unique packaging or product benefit. However, in the process of selecting products for this study there were two out of the five brands that lacked any obvious innovation when I made the purchases. This provided an edge for those brands that did demonstrate innovation and only reinforced what the interviewees felt about the two brand images earlier on in conversation on that topic.

My first sample was Maybelline Fit Me Foundation and Falsies Mascara, two new products introduced to market. The goal was to understand if the Fit Me packaging evolution would alter the current younger less expensive image of Maybelline among the interviewees. The second product, Falsies Mascara, was selected to understand if the name of the product was a positive one for women. The following is how women felt about both product and packaging innovations.

Fit Me Foundation with its strong sleek black packaging begins to move the Maybelline brand equity to a more sophisticated place. However, women saw the packaging as a disconnection from the Maybelline image in their minds. They did react favorably to the technological story of self-adjusting to ones skin tone. This was driven purely by the products name. Women referred to it as more "classy" and "something that one would be proud to pull out of your purse" product. They recognized the brand's effort to go "more upscale", however, with this came some criticism about brand continuity. Women thought that it looked like a completely different brand, even department store level, and felt that while it was incongruous for Maybelline it was an attempt to appeal to a new audience.

Falsies Mascara from Maybelline on the other hand evoked a very different reaction. The name and color palette was polarizing to women mostly driven by their age. Younger interviewees liked it and older women did not. The name was seen as something that would make your lashes look "fake". The color palette was referred to as "cheap" looking. Younger women did see the humor in the name and said it was something they would try. When asked about its relationship to Maybelline women agreed that Falsies Mascara was more in keeping with their impression of the brand.

I found it interesting that while one product, Fit Me Foundation, could evolve Maybelline from a younger and less expensive image in a positive way, Falsies Mascara, launched months earlier only reinforced it. The take away among the majority of the women was that Falsies Mascara was synergistic with their impression of the Maybelline brand and it reminded them of Great Lash Mascara, an older Maybelline product.

The majority of the women stated that the Fit Me product was far more sophisticated than the products they have come to associate with Maybelline. To them the brand impression begins to shift to a more modern and upscale product. While they saw this evolution as a brand improvement they also felt it was inconsistent with the current Maybelline image they remembered.

Next fresh out of my Ziploc bag was Cover Girl. The two products chosen had very different product innovation stories. One product was Simply Ageless, a foundation with Olay moisturizer added to it. The other was a new product from Cover Girl called NatureLuxe.

In the exploration of the two products and innovation, the goal was to find out if the addition of the Olay moisturizer in the Cover Girl Simply Ageless Foundation added any value. In the case of

NatureLuxe it was whether a brand like Cover Girl could capitalize on the "all natural" ingredient trend that was building momentum in the beauty world.

Here is what I found out about the two.

Simply Ageless Foundation with the addition of Olay's moisturizer was seen as a 'do more for me', and, 'more bang for the buck' product but questions arose as to how effective the product benefit really was. Interviewees felt it was a good value and that it would be something that women with busy lives would use. Convenience of having the two benefits in one seemed to be a good idea for the majority of the women. A second positive about the product was the idea of not having to layer a lot of product on your face.

For women below the age of twenty-five the idea was polarizing given the specific images they had of Cover Girl and Olay. Cover Girl was for a younger woman and Olay for a more mature one. If there was any positive for the women in this demographic it was Olay's credibility. The following quote sums it up. "It's weird, Cover Girl is younger and not concerned with aging while Olay is my mother's brand."

The second product from Cover Girl was NatureLuxe. This new product struck a cord with younger women given its implied natural proposition. However, upon closer inspection, women started to wonder just how natural it really was. In addition, women were concerned that a more natural approach to foundation would cost more. The plastic packaging also seemed to contradict the idea of 'natural'. Implying natural, and actually being natural, created greater skepticism over the product's overall proposition. This point-of-view was both from a packaging and ingredient perspective. Some of the women thought that it was most likely the "same old product in a different package", acknowledging that it was smart marketing for today's health trend. The following interviewee summed up the overall take on this product innovation.

"I have seen this. I noticed it because I am prone to look for more natural stuff with fewer chemicals in the formula but I didn't think this was any different. I looked at the list of ingredients, most of which I cannot pronounce. I don't care about luxury if I am buying a natural product, I care about the natural part."

The same interviewee went on to say. "Luxury and nature are compatible; it is a luxury to be able to buy natural products. Like juice. Pomegranate juice is natural, it's not luxury pomegranate. The luxury is built into the natural. When you look at the ingredients there are very few elements that are natural. It really looks more like marketing and less like innovation."

After reviewing the two Cover Girl product innovations I learned that Simply Ageless with Olay was seen as a good value given the 2 in 1 nature of the technology, that being foundation and skin care. However this combination created an issue for the interviewees as to whom the target is. This question was driven by the strong brand images of Cover Girl and Olay and the different age groups the two brands appealed to. Even with the two positives mentioned about the Simply Ageless Foundation innovation, the majority of women said they would not be interested in it. They did think that for "someone other than them it was a good value" because of the combination of the two brands.

NatureLuxe seemed to be a bigger issue among the interviewees. The platform of natural implied by the product name and packaging cues created skepticism among most of the women. There was also little to no connection between NatureLuxe and Cover Girl in terms of equity value. Adding to the lack of product credibility based on packaging and ingredients, women saw no connection to the Cover Girl brand they were familiar with. In a recent store check I was unable to locate NatureLuxe on the shelf. This leads me to believe it has been discontinued.

Unzipping the next bag I placed L'Oreal Paris products on the table. L'Oreal Paris's product superiority was already mentioned by the majority of the interviewees earlier on in the interviews as a big part of the brand's reputation. Known for its innovation in both product and packaging it was easy to select two products that provided strong propositions to get women to react to. The first to be discussed was a foundation, True Match Roller with its unique application tool. The second was L'Oreal Paris Lash Boosting Serum and Mascara for its advanced technology for the mass market.

True Match Roller is a roll on foundation that did evoke interest among all the interviewees given its application system. The tool for applying the makeup resembles a miniature paint roller and upon further inspection either intrigued or humored them. The concern with this product was the possible "flatness" of the application on the skin and the issue they may have using the roller on the curvy parts around their noses.

"I've never seen anything like this but I think the roll on might make the application challenging. My issue is with contouring the face using a paint roller."

Some of the interviewees reinforced the "paint roller" connection in a more positive way. They felt that it was a really "cool" way to apply the foundation. This included speed and not messy. "I have never seen this before but in theory it is smart with an even application and it's portable." Women who were not concerned about the paint roller idea saw it as a cleaner way to apply foundation. The positive take was that it would go on smooth and would not leave marks, which is a concern among the majority of interviewees who did use a foundation.

The second product, L'Oreal Paris Lash Boosting Serum and Mascara, was the most innovative product that I had among all the brands in this section of the study. As L'Oreal Paris does best, it looks to prestige and specialty product innovation for inspiration then replicates them for the mass market at an affordable price point. In this second innovation example L'Oreal Paris borrowed from the world of pharmaceuticals.

Latisse, the source of inspiration for L'Oreal Paris, requires a doctor's prescription. The lash product is prescribed for women with inadequate or thin lashes. The benefit of this product is to grow lashes so they are longer and fuller. Latisse had been on the market for a little over a year when L'Oreal Paris launched a version of this product that did not require a prescription. You may recall the Latisse advertising with Brook Shields that quickly built awareness of the product and its benefit. It was also good timing on L'Oreal's part to capitalize on the heavy media and promotional investment that Allergan, the pharmaceutical company that owns Latisse, made in educating consumers about this new technology.

The L'Oreal Lash Boosting Serum was first met with skepticism among the women interviewed but upon further evaluation a strong willingness to try emerged. The desire to try the product was driven mostly by the recall of Latisse.

Innovative packaging with a clinical feel for Lash Boosting Serum enhanced product credibility. Interviewees referred to this product as an affordable alternative and the added bonus of not having to get a prescription from a doctor—"Seems simple and more natural". The interest was driven by individual need or desire for longer lashes. Mimicking an established pharmaceutical product was seen as appropriate given L'Oreal Paris's equity in product innovation.

L'Oreal Paris maintains a very strong equity of quality and performance among the women interviewed which made both product innovations a natural fit to the brand. However, what consistently emerged form the interviewees that primarily purchased products at mass was cost. In some cases women said they weren't surprised by the advanced technology in both benefit and application that the two products demonstrated. In regard to purchasing either product, the final consideration would be the cost. This group made the sentiment of affordability very clear when it came to the "cost" of these two unique product innovations from L'Oreal Paris. For women who only shopped at mass, the price point of L'Oreal Paris was in most cases a bit too expensive for them. For those interviewees that were department store shopper cost was not a consideration.

The fourth brand in the discussion on product innovation was Revlon. As mentioned earlier I was aware of Revlon's recent advances. While its evolution was the buzz of the beauty world, the interviewees had not been exposed to it, so the older image of the brand would be their only frame of reference for the interview. This might also explain why there was very little in the form of product innovation when I selected my samples. The brand may have been waiting for the new advertising to launch in support of the new product introductions. The need for a brand intervention was timely given the predominate question during the interviews: "What has Revlon done lately?"

Revlon products presented lacked any innovation, which only reinforced the perception the women already had of the brand. The women could only reference the familiar red nail polish and lip color and the two products presented, eye shadow and lipstick, offered no product news. With little to work with I presented two products for the interviewees to consider.

The eye shadow 'quad' (as the 4 shades in a compact are called) generated some conversation among the interviewees that focused on the likeability of the 4 colors. As for the lipstick they felt the packaging was "sleek and professional". The interviewees then reverted back to talking about what they knew of the brand, repeating what they had said earlier about the brands faded past.

All the women interviewed associated the color red with this brand. Celebrity is not an element that was obvious to them. Lacking an innovation story, Revlon's strongest equity is in lip and nail. Women could not see beyond it being an "older" brand. It was mostly referred to as "the brand my mother used."

The brand equity is seen as lower end in mass, on par with Cover Girl but slightly above Maybelline. Innovation was not mentioned. Most women felt that with this brand it was pretty much the "same old thing" and with that the interviewees felt that it had little to no point of competitive difference.

The discussion of Revlon did not generate any excitement or interest. It was difficult to provide any stimulus that would change women's overall feeling of what the brand had done lately. Over the past couple of years, Revlon's brand look was moving away from its black and gold heritage. It was becoming more modern and using brighter color pallets. Even the brand logo has been revised to create a more contemporary look. The brand renovation is also supported by the addition of Emma Stone, a young actress who is smart, approachable and beautiful. What the interviewees were responding to in our interviews was the images they had of an older brand-proving once again that timing is everything.

The last in the line up of beauty brands was Avon. Upon handing out the Avon catalogue at the beginning of each interview I quickly learned that it did not create much enthusiasm among the women. If there was any innovation across the beauty products featured it went unnoticed given the clutter on every page. With this understanding

I realized that on the topic of product innovation I might be better off with a different approach in regard to Avon.

In my beauty experience I've always embraced the corporate mission for Avon (not to mention my new found loyalty to Genevieve in Harlem). For me this included three elements:

1. Avon, a company of women for women.
2. Avon's extensive global sales force 6 million+, made up primarily of women.
3. Avon's association with supporting the fight against breast cancer.

These three points separated Avon as a beauty brand from all the others. But the point of the conversation was to find out if it had the same impact on women in the study. So I asked. Surprisingly the awareness of the three elements was relatively low among the women I interviewed. The strongest of the three that the interviewees referenced was Avon's association with breast cancer awareness. Women did feel that the company was doing "good" with this association but in the end it didn't guarantee product purchase. It did make them feel better about the company but they were more interested in the quality of Avon products. In addition to concerns about product quality, they were not sure how much of the "give back" was real. They questioned whether it was just a marketing ploy to get them to buy. "I don't know how much they are giving to the 'cause'; they may be just slapping it on the product to get me to buy it."

Ultimately it was made very clear by the women that any interest in purchasing product was tied to performance and not to philanthropy. "I don't know how much a difference it [philanthropy] would make at the end of the day when I am buying a product. No animal testing is more important to me."

I found it rather interesting the way women talked about the separation between causes and selling products. Having been a big advocate of brand give back and the support of causes, I was hearing first hand the skepticism that existed on the relationship between philanthropy and marketing. Many women mentioned that beauty brands were in the business of selling products and not supporting causes. Enlightened by the lack of interest among the women on the topic of those three equity elements, I then asked what the women thought about the Avon catalogue.

The unanimous consensus was that the catalogue was overwhelming and that Avon was diluting its beauty equity with so many offerings. The catalogue was seen as a bit cluttered and thus hard to shop. There were a few women that liked the idea of taking time to shop the catalogue. I think the best comment on this was in the form of a question. "Why do they sell more than beauty products? I'd rather they just be beauty experts".

The catalogue diversity of products created confusion among the interviewees. "I guess by putting their name on it helps to sell other things, but it gets a little blurry on what they stand for".

The general consensus was best summed up by one of the women:

"I don't object to all this stuff, I just wonder if their beauty products are really effective".

What I ultimately learned from the interviewees did not surprise me given my own impression of the brand based on the catalogue and the products that I had in hand. The brand did appear to be all over the place and product innovation was lacking. What did surprise me were the responses, or lack of that the interviewees had about the three elements that I thought separated Avon from the other beauty brands. Given those unique points I expected more of the women to rally behind a company with women as their focus but it seemed that these elements were not strong enough to guarantee a purchase. What was essential to the interviewees was product performance.

The insights on product innovation garnered from the women in the interviews were straightforward. It was at this point that I confirmed the fine line that exists between marketers and consumers when it comes to evaluating actual products. From a marketing perspective it is all about telling a product story that will entice consumers to consider purchasing. From the consumer angle it is about a clear understanding of what purpose the product benefit will serve. Setting aside the aesthetics of packaging, color and scent, women insist on understanding how the product will work and simply what it will do for them.

It was evident from the five brands selected for this that L'Oreal Paris, Cover Girl and Maybelline offered varying degrees of innovation. Revlon and Avon did not, but as mentioned earlier, Revlon was in the early stages of their makeover unlike Avon who offered a variety of products beyond beauty, which resulted in a lack of credibility among the interviewees.

The interviewees confirmed that L'Oreal Paris was the leader in innovation, both in beauty benefits and interesting application systems, such as the roll on foundation. The brand's value was further enhanced by the technology behind the Lash Booster product given the familiarity that the women had with the prescription version, Lattisse. Both products were consistent with how women felt about the L'Oreal image; however both products contributed to the feeling among the women that while it maintains a high standard of quality the brand is more expensive.

How the interviewees felt about Cover Girl's product samples was different than that of L'Oreal Paris. To them the Simply Ageless Foundation with the addition of Olay seemed to be a contradiction. The legacy of Olay among the women as "my mom's brand", as an ingredient in Cover Girl (a much younger brand), seemed to be a disconnection among the interviewees. The question raised is: can the equity of one brand add credibility even if its target audience of women is considerably different?

For the interviewees, Cover Girl's NatureLuxe suffered from a credibility issue. For the women in the study it simply came down to brand messaging and being honest. Implying one thing and being something else, among the younger women, raise red flags in terms of brand transparency. "Natural should have packaging and formulas that are truly natural, not plastic containers and all these chemical ingredients."

Maybelline's sample of product innovation revealed a different type of insight on brand evolution. Here the two products on display conjured up a feeling that they were not from the same company. While Falsies Mascara had a young and flirtatious feel, Fit Me Foundation had a sleek and sophisticated vibe. The brand's evolution may be similar to that of Revlon. In regard to real product or benefit innovation, neither product demonstrated any uniqueness; rather, the innovation was perceived to be superficial. "Nothing new with either of these two products. Looks more like a packaging thing than anything else."

In this section of the interviews the third lesson was the importance of packaging and product innovation as key drivers to purchasing. Women were emphatic that brands whose labels clearly communicated product benefit held an advantage over those that did not. If the brand does not provided any new value either in its packaging or product innovation, as in the case of Revlon, it was considered a "same old thing" brand.

In their evaluation of the products the interviewees broke it down in a few simple thoughts.

1. What makes this product better than the next one?
2. If it's new and improved, will it cost more?
3. If I don't quickly understand what it does, I'm not interested in it.

Finally, and mostly driven by the conversation about Avon, brand causes were recognized as a good thing overall. However, questions were raised about the authenticity of the partnership between the brand and the cause. Queries such as "how much does the company actually donate?" and "are they doing this just to make me feel better about the brand?" were common. The additional insight gleaned from the interviewees was a brand cause on its own is not enough to promote sales. What mattered most to the interviewees was that it was a good product that addressed their needs. Brand cause came second.

Lather. Rinse. Repeat.

Hair care is a category where the selection of a product can be influenced by packaging, scent and most of all, trial and error. It is the beauty segment where women are always on the look out for the "one" that works. This consumer behavior is primarily driven by the overpromises made by the beauty brands and a belief that over time a shampoo stops working. Neutrogena built an entire brand based on this insight of switching products after fourteen days to remove the build up residue from your regular shampoo. The simple truth is that a hair care product can temporarily alter the quality of one's hair but not change it long term.

Early in the development of this category, shampoos and conditioners basic function was to clean and condition hair. The product offerings were simple back when you could select versions for dry, oily, fine, normal, anti-dandruff, and color treated hair types. Today brand offerings have evolved from hair type to a selection of benefits that include strengthening, smoothing, frizz control, sleeking, volumizing, highlighting, nourishing, anti-breakage, and more recently age defying (even though it's a scientific fact that hair is dead)!

Before we get to what interviewees had to say about the various hair products in the study let's look back at some of the more memorable hair care brands and how the category has evolved.

In the early days of hair care advertising it was a matter of lather, rinse and repeat. Rather simple instructions to achieve the typical end benefit of beautiful hair. In the 70's and 80's the advertising theme for hair care was a world of girl gets boy with a flip of her locks. Male appreciation was an executional element used in brand communications - most of the time in the form of a hand caressing a woman's hair. Soft to the touch, shiny hair and fluid movements were the visual cues of beauty. The scent of the product was and still is a key product driver in purchasing, as in the example of Herbal Essences in the early 70's. It's not uncommon to see women removing the cap from a product to smell the scent while standing in the store aisle. Like the scent of the product, packaging is a strong consideration for purchasing. In the late 80's, while I was working on Vidal Sassoon, I heard a number of women in a focus group remark how they liked to leave the brown cylinder shaped bottles out in their bathrooms for friends and guests to notice.

Women today are always searching for the one shampoo that works the best for them and rarely are they satisfied for long as some of the interviewees in this study confirm. Salon related products were not that prevalent at mass during this time, but it wasn't long before they arrived on the scene.

Currently there are a number of salon brands being sold at mass. In the past they were only sold in salons that upheld their exclusivity.

Two salon brands that entered the mass market early on were Nexxus and Vidal Sassoon. Vidal Sassoon, the first celebrity stylist, attempted to position itself as the salon expert at mass while Nexxus made its mass debut with a conditioning product called Humectress in the mid 80's. Both had extended their distribution from salons and subsequently were looked down upon by professional stylists.

A pivotal moment in the mass hair care evolution was the introduction of Unilever's Salon Selectives. The unique proposition they offered was a form of customization in the hair care segment. While there was no real association with a salon other than the name and slogan; "Like you just walked out of the salon" (recently the slogan for Suave, another Unilever brand), the product lineup stepped outside of the status quo in hair care. The product options for women extended beyond the typical dry, normal, and fine versions of care to a matrix of products based on benefit and not hair type. For example, a woman could select a volumizing shampoo and pair it with a frizz control conditioner. This mix and match approach to selecting product was the first form of personalization in hair care. It allowed women to choose a shampoos and conditioner based on personal need.

Another influential product introduction in hair care was the launch of the 2-in-1-hair care technology derived from a silicone formula developed by Proctor & Gamble. This new formulation allowed cleansing and conditioning to coexist in one bottle and it was called Pert Plus. The technology developed by Proctor & Gamble appeared on the market in 1987. The proposition of hair care convenience was the core message with visuals reflecting the more active unisex lifestyles of the day. Proctor & Gamble soon after applied the same technology to Pantene. This move revitalized Pantene and by adding Pro V, (Pro Vitamin), to its name and it became the gold standard for healthier hair. Within a few years the brand became a global leader in hair care. It was also the first time that health was part of the beauty care vernacular in hair care. Shine was the new measurement for healthy hair and the slogan "So healthy it shines" was born. Yes, there was now a variety of benefits that one could obtain from a bottle beyond clean hair!

With this brief chronology of the evolution of hair care let us move on to the interviews. I had selected a variety of hair care brands for various reasons starting with salon brands. Here I wanted to explore how the interviewees viewed the relationship between price and quality associated with salon brands sold in the mass market.

When discussing the relationship between salon brands and price value with the interviewees I presented them with two brands, TRESemme and Nexxus. The women first saw the lower priced brand, TRESemme, as the better value. When asked about which brand was a better quality product they unanimously switched their choice to Nexxus. This simple exercise demonstrated that the women interviewed were able to separate product quality from dollar value. In essence, the age-old belief that you get what you pay for was validated.

"I would go with Nexxus. I don't look at the price and know that TRESemme is a cheap big bottle and I would rather have one that works…you have this conversation with yourself at the shelf every time."

The interviewees who were salon brand users were buying their products at the salon, and, for the most part, it was because of stylist recommendation.

Among all the women interviewed, while price mattered, it was product performance that was more important. If they found a product that worked best on their hair that was the one they were using. The women had a great deal of experience with the salon segment, since they were always trying new shampoos that promised the benefit they were looking to achieve. The level of product satisfaction would vary from woman to woman and each of them was willing to consider the latest offering if they thought it would deliver on its promise.

In general, the interviewees believed that salon brands do maintain a halo of better quality within the hair care segment. Price and value are part of the segment dynamics and better product performance is expected from higher price brands. Large quantities of salon product at lower prices create skepticism, but obviously are seen as a better dollar value.

It is a known fact that hair care brands are constantly looking for "news value" to attract users. Often this is done with an ingredient story. A unique ingredient tied to a benefit is one way of capturing the consumer's attention in a "big, better, different" way. Next in the study was to discuss with the interviewees how new ingredients in a selection of hair care brands influenced their impression of the brands. The interviewees were given three brands to evaluate.

The first shampoo was L'Oreal's EverStrong Sulfate Free Formula. Here, it was the lack of sulfates that sparked favorable comments. The positive here was that it contained less chemicals, however, the interviewees wondered what the sulfates in a shampoo did and what was in the formula to replace it.

The interviewees asked if the product would deliver on clean given that sulfates were removed. While they thought it might be better for them they quickly talked about what difference it would really make given that many of them referred to the hard water containing iron and other minerals that they had at home. In the end the women felt that the lack of chemical in any product used on the body would be a good thing, even for the few interviewees that had no idea what the sulfates in a shampoo did. The primary role of sulfates in a shampoo is to create that "luxurious lather" we have all come to expect and enjoy.

The fact is that sulfates in a shampoo can alter or strip the color out of color treated hair. The technology for the L'Oreal Paris product was inspired by a high-end salon brand called Pureology.

The second shampoo ingredient example was Garnier's Fructis Fortifying Shampoo with olive, shea and avocado oils. The interviewees found the 'oils' in the product acceptable, especially for conditioning purposes. Those that were not interested in the brand said so because they did not know which type of hair the product worked best on given the three oils that were on the label. These women quickly dismissed any possible consideration to try the product. What became a greater discussion in regard to the Fructis product had little to do with the "oils" and more about the color of the green packaging that the interviewees found to be objectionable.

Consistent among the interviewees at this point was a growing skepticism regarding ingredients and the product's ability to deliver on its promise. The majority of the women stated that they have "heard it all" regarding hair care brands that claim "New and Improved" based on a new ingredient. As one interviewee lamented all of the new ingredient stories were "a dime a dozen". "Every brand is trying to seduce you with the latest and greatest new thing." Another interviewee said that the "New and Improved" aspect with shampoos was just another way to get you "to buy more". "Why did they have to improve it if in the past they said it was so great for you?"

The third hair care example in the context of ingredient was Herbal Essences Body Envy Passion Fruit and Pearl Fusion shampoo.

The interviewees thought that the idea of "fusion of passion fruit and pearl " to be silly, but felt that it was in keeping with both the packaging and the youthful image of the brand. There were a number of interviewees that remembered the former Herbal Essences packaging and scent. A few of the women referenced the advertising inspired by the scene in "When Harry met Sally" where Meg Ryan dramatically fakes an orgasm while sitting in a deli on the lower East side of New York. Herbal Essence used this idea as a humorous way to communicate the brands sensorial equity.

On the topic of shampoo ingredients the interviewees were not inspired by the three examples provided. In general, the topic of shampoo did not spark much enthusiasm for the majority of interviewees. This lack of excitement was primarily driven by the frustration and disappointment by the interviewees when the brands promises did not live up to the hype. In essence the ingredient stories only underscored the skepticism the interviewees have about product performance.

The learning from this part of the study was that, on the topic of hair care, the interviewees fell into two distinct camps: the Loyalist and the Seeker.

Regardless of salon equity or innovative ingredients, if a woman has found the "one" that works for her hair she becomes fiercely loyal to the brand. The interviewees stated that when loyal to a particular brand she would travel with it for fear of not being able to find it upon her arrival. The Loyalist is also the one who becomes the brands best advocate given her enthusiasm for having found a shampoo that "delivers on its promise". Most of the interviewees in this study have found their preferred hair care product by way of a recommendation from a friend or their stylist. In the case of a stylist recommendation, the women in my study said that once an expert told them which salon product to use they would never consider going back to a mass shampoo brand.

The second camp is the interviewee who is switching from brand to brand in pursuit of the one that works. Most of these women were shopping at mass for their shampoo products. Her constant trial and error approach is mostly driven by the disappointment she experiences from brands that do not deliver on their promise.

In hair care the reality is that brands that promise benefits including volume or smooth results are unachievable with some hair types. For example, a woman with fine and thin hair is not going to see volume without products with a wax ingredient for thickening. For a woman with curly hair looking for a smooth look, she has three ways to achieve it: a hair iron, a blow dryer, or a "Japanese Treatment", also known as thermal reconditioning at a salon. The results will not come from a bottle. If you are born with curly hair you will need to straighten it to get it smooth and if you have straight hair and you are dreaming of curls you will need to get a curling iron or a perm. Ouch!

With continuous expansion of the hair care category-new brands and benefits-women will always be tempted to try and hope that maybe she will find one that really works for her. The search is part of the category dynamic and for some of the women it is a never ending one. Women look at their hair care needs differently as they get older. Most of the older interviewees in the group preferred to keep their hair short for that 'wash and go' convenience. The hair care category is a multi-billion dollar business that continues to discover new stories for women to believe in and buy into. The fact remains that DNA has a lot to do with the type and quality of your hair. Styling, weaves and extensions can influence how your hair looks but at the end of the day you pretty much have to work with what mom and dad gave you.

Dove shampoo was part of the exploration on hair care. However, the overwhelming conversation among the interviewees quickly moved from product performance to the Dove "Real Beauty" proposition which deserves its very own chapter given its impact and scope.

Bar Soap and
Real Beauty

The Dove shampoo product was selected in order to understand if its strong equities as a bar soap could translate to a hair care line. Not surprisingly, women's impressions of this brand were overshadowed by its "Real Beauty" campaign. Focusing on the question of soap and hair care the women in the group had mixed feelings.

"I use Dove soap, but would not be inclined to use the shampoo".

From another woman:

"I have not used this. I think of it [Dove] as a soap only".

Most of the women interviewed held Dove soap in high regard. Many recalled the ¼ moisturizing cream as part of its brand equity. While others saw it as quality bar soap they didn't see bar soap equities readily transferred to hair care; rather they saw the equity more in body care. Beyond these points, women did not have much to say about the products. Interestingly, the conversation nearly always shifted from the products to Dove's "Real Beauty" campaign. The campaign created an empowerment platform for Dove and it continues to be part of their marketing strategy.

From my own recall of this campaign I remember the anticipation within the beauty industry that something big was coming from the Dove brand. There were early reports about the brands "new approach" in beauty. My first encounter with it was upon landing at Narita Airport in Tokyo. The airport terminal was plastered with Dove banners, no copy that I recall, just the iconic white Dove against the blue. This campaign was the prelude to approaching beauty care in an entirely different way.

As mentioned earlier the Dove Real Beauty campaign made its debut in 2004 based on global research conducted in multiple countries. Dove reached out to over thirty-two hundred women to better understand current perceptions of beauty. Of the thirty-two hundred women in the study only two percent considered themselves to be beautiful. This staggering statistic led to the crusade to change women's definition/perception of beauty.

There has been a lot written about the Dove Real Beauty effort both from its critics and those who consider it a financial success. The campaign continues to be part of their communications plan even today. "Sketches", the current expression of Dove's empowerment campaign, launched in 2012. The tactic was simply to highlight how women describe themselves, which is then captured by a sketch artist. The same exercise is repeated except this time the subject's physical characteristics are described by a person each woman has met for the first time. This person proceeds to describe, to the artist only, how they see the subject's characteristics and attributes.

Both sketches are shown to the subject at the end of the session and reveal that the sketched subject has a very different visual impression of herself, which is mostly negative than the stranger who describes her to the same artist. The take away from this exercise is clear. Women tend to be critical of their looks and internalize their perceived flaws. As a nod to Dove this may be the result of a judgmental beauty world. I do think that as part of the internalization women tend to focus on their flaws—large nose, thin hair, weak lips, etc. When a complete stranger is describing the woman to the artist what she sees is the total composition and not the individual parts. What she describes is far more positive and true to what the woman being sketched really looks like. In this case I do believe that Dove succeeds in its effort to expose misaligned impressions women have of themselves. Perhaps this misalignment is guided by unattainable standards in beauty. It is also rooted in basic insecurities of women on which Dove capitalizes.

The Dove "Real Beauty" campaign created a great deal of interest among women given its message of individuality and beauty. While I embrace the idea of this inclusiveness, I have to wonder if in their approach there exists an element of manipulation.

Contrary to what some may initially see, the "Real Beauty" campaign is not unlike most advertising in the beauty world. It's a marketing strategy that leverages extensive research and the singular insight that women believe there is an unrealistic idea of beauty that one can achieve. I believe what Dove did in its campaign approach was to capitalize on women's insecurities by reminding them of this "unattainable" beauty. What Dove did in the process was to establish itself as a beauty brand. Up until this campaign, Dove's image was that of a bar soap. Now entering the hair care segment it needed to do more than leverage it's bar soap equity in a unique way. What resulted created a disruption in the category with its philosophy on beauty. The "Real Beauty" campaign was considered a major success in establishing Dove as a beauty brand by challenging the existing codes of beauty providing the brand with a distinct and relevant voice.

There are two elements regarding the "Real Beauty" campaign that are problematic.

The first is already well documented by the critics of this campaign. On one side was the empowerment factor of the "Real Beauty" message for all women and on the other side was an Axe deodorant campaign, targeted to men, objectifying women as sex objects. The question among the critics was how could the same company-Unilever -promote opposing images of women? Women who are aware of Unilever's Axe deodorant campaign that was running at the same time as the Dove women empowerment campaign considered it hypocritical and became vocal about it.

U.S. News reporter Danielle Kurtzleben, in response to the Dove's "Sketches" campaign, writes; "Dove continues its campaign to bolster women's self esteem, yet it finds itself continually besieged by questions about internal contradictions. Many have pointed out for years that Dove's message of promoting women's body images conflicts with ads from Axe, a male-oriented toiletry brand owned by Dove's parent company, Unilever. In addition, critics say that Dove's ads contradict themselves, taking aim at the beauty industry while shilling beauty products."

The second element is my own elaboration on what Danielle Kurzleben mentions in her comments about "taking aim at the beauty industry while shilling beauty products". In my opinion Dove had questionable credibility in its attempt to define beauty standards simply because it is not a comprehensive beauty brand. Dove operates on the lowest end of beauty transformation and engagement within the industry. Once a bar soap only, now into hair care and body washes, the products provide little in terms of transformative beauty when compared to cosmetics, skin care and hair color. Perhaps if Dove competed in those beauty segments its "Real Beauty" message would signal a different tone and approach.

I completely understand the current 'image retouching' and 'runway thin' debates, but beauty is about empowerment through enhancement. While Dove featured a variety of women in its campaigns the women I interviewed appreciated it but they did not aspire to be one of them. What they did appreciate was the refreshing approach to the beauty conversation and a recognition that beauty comes in all shapes and sizes. "Real women, like me", was the sticking point, but when asked if they wanted to be seen in that way, all of the interviewees said "No".

I probed further on the "Real Beauty" campaign to listen to what women had to say about it:

"I have used Dove shampoo, I love the real women campaign. I thought it tapped into what women are looking for, more real women and less Hollywood."

"It [Real Beauty] reached out to a lot of women, it was refreshing."

"I remember an ad with women wearing wigs and a lot of full size models, be who you are idea. A good thing but I didn't buy any products."

What I had heard among the women suggested that Dove made a strong point, but it didn't motivate them to aspire to be like the Dove women featured in the advertising.

Women talked about how controversial the un-retouched photography was, referencing "real butts and freckles on the faces", but many said it did not inspire them to want to look beautiful. Most interesting was that this "realness factor" only motivated one interviewee in this study to have purchased the product.

The focus on real women was entirely just that. In the advertising there were no product demonstrations or dramatic beauty shots, just every day women of all ages, shapes and sizes. One example of the advertising featured a fifty plus female with long grey hair. The copy in the ad asked the reader to select if the woman was grey or gorgeous with a line of copy that read, "Why can't more women feel glad to be Grey? Join the beauty debate." The campaign for Real Beauty was meant to create a debate about the unrealistic beauty standards expressed by a majority of the thirty-two hundred women in their study. At the same time that the Real Beauty campaign was running, Dove promoted products with traditional advertising. This approach featured Dove products and comparisons to competitive shampoos and conditioners in an effort to communicate Dove's product superiority. They did not use fashion models in these executions, only hand models, whose faces were never seen, holding product packaging.

Many in the interviews mentioned that they did not think the products were quality products. They respected the campaigns honesty but the lack of transformation was obvious to them. Women are very wary when it comes to brand messaging and if the message only makes them feel good without providing relevance for the product usage, their take away is that "it made me feel good" but it did not translate into a product sale.

In the context of beauty products, the interviewees talked about the importance of the transformative power of a beauty product, the importance of seeing the "before and after"—the effect the benefit provides. The basis of the "Real Beauty" campaign was attitudinal and not a real demonstration of the transformative power of product even though they attempted to convey product superiority in the alternate product only advertising.

On the topic of "Real Beauty", women said that they like to see that even celebrities are women that have problems just like them. The transformation provides a relatable situation and product credibility. The acne related product Pro-Active was noted as a great example of providing celebrity transformation with great credibility.

All in all, the general feeling among all the individuals was that beauty companies were out of touch with women, sometime pushing it too far with retouching. This thought aligned with what Dove and the "real beauty" campaign attempted to achieve. The women interviewed still hoped that beauty companies would "wake up" and realize that today's woman lives in a "real world".

In the end, while other beauty companies zig, Dove's zag to the other end of the beauty standard spectrum was meant to underscore insecurities and vulnerabilities that come from living in a highly commercial world driven by luxury images of "la dolce vita", (the sweet life).

Another positive aspect about the Dove campaign is its effort to showcase diversity in terms of both body type and ethnicity. This effort, which was the core of the 2004 work, was a reminder that we are not all the same and that our individuality should be recognized and celebrated. It is this singular element that is the strength of the campaign. It is interesting to note, too, that it wasn't until 1997 that L'Oreal featured its first African American spokesperson, Vanessa Williams, in print and television advertising in the US. Viva la diversity...

The discussion on "Real Beauty" with the women reminded me of something I had heard years ago from Myrna Blyth, the former editor-in-chief and publishing director of Ladies Home Journal. She observed, "Too many women today think that it's okay to run around looking good enough. Well, I think it's time that women start thinking 'good enough isn't good enough'!"

Myrna shared this thought with me over breakfast many years ago and I have used it as a standard of measurement in my own life. I find it interesting that the core of its meaning is not about holding to a set standard of beauty, but rather it is holding to a set standard of being at ones best at all times. While the beauty industry may suggest a certain unattainable level of beauty, its intent is to inspire every woman to reach beyond and discover hidden potential that may lie within. It is the motivation to look your very best that I find lacking in the Dove Real Beauty campaign. Yes, of course, the power of self-acceptance is very important, but what the beauty industry tries to do goes beyond self-acceptance-to discovery and self-expression.

There is no doubt that Dove attempted to debunk the beauty myths of the Western world. "Real Beauty" challenged all of us in the industry to take notice and to evaluate our communications and approach to diversity. The campaign was also addressing the changes in the world around us. The important shift in beauty standards now being replaced by individuality that is underscored with a generation of women now with body piercing and tattoos. The new standards of beauty are accelerated by the global access that the Internet provides. Self-expression, personalization and information are becoming the new elements of beauty making the idea of Dove's "Real Beauty" almost as dated as the former standard of beauty it was trying to uproot.

Skin Deep

A t my last count there were 3,188 products available on the Walmart website. This includes everything from exfoliators to sun care. Once you have navigated the number of choices you can also compare prices. Of the twenty beauty brands listed on the site the skin care product price points range from $1.97 for a 13 oz tub of Walmart's Equate 100% Pure Petroleum Jelly Skin Protectant used for dry skin to an anti-aging cream called Radiance New York Time Machine Ultimate Youth that contains Temple Viper Snake Venom (?!) 1.7 ounces that sells for $139.99. Of course this may be seen as a great value when compared to La Mer's Creame de la Mer 16.5 ounces sold in department stores for $2000.

At mass the skin care segment is beginning to tier itself similar to that in hair care with low, medium and premium pricing. The premium pricing categories are now competing with the department store brands. Olay had been on a campaign strategy for years comparing their brand to department store brands at a fraction of the cost. The campaign has recently been replaced with "Your Best Beautiful" featuring Katie Holmes. Perhaps it is because they own a growing brand in the prestige category called SKII. L'Oreal, with its multiple prestige lines in specialty and department stores, has never attempted to compare their mass brands to prestige brands.

Once you have scouted the selection and reviewed pricing, there is the ingredient list to consider. When it comes to skin care moisturizers that are used to soften and smooth skin there are on average five commonly used ingredients. Helping to provide hydration for your skin by holding water are glycerin and hyaluronic acid. There is sodium hyaluronate which also holds water and shea butter that moisturizes. The last is vitamin E that acts as an antioxidant. The list of ingredients grows even longer when we look at anti-aging products. Today the range of common to unique skin care ingredients for wrinkle repair can include; pro-retinol, hydroxyl acid, calcium, grape seed, collagen, vitamin C, B, B12, placenta and perhaps unicorn dust just to mention a few.

Of all the beauty segments, skin care is the most confusing. That is why most women seek out answers on the Internet or, for those that can, department stores sales people. Interviewees, even those who buy their skin care products at mass, think that the sales person is one of the best sources for skin care information. The department store sales force is the person that often provides consumer education. This one-to-one service as well as better quality packaging translates into a higher mark-up on department store beauty products.

When we look at two of the major players in today's mass skincare market we turn to Procter & Gamble's Olay and L'Oreal Paris.

Both companies have tiered their portfolios based on pricing, age segment, and degree of intervention/repair. Both companies have products on the market that address aging skin. These products promise you can look good at any age. With this in mind I talked with the interviewees in my study to understand what influenced them in the area of skin care.

In general, the interviewees I spoke to all shared the same feeling that they are more aware of the need to take care of their skin—despite diverse demographics. Even the younger women in the study were concerned about sun damage and early intervention to help prevent lines and wrinkles from forming. These interviewees were mainly influenced by their moms whom they say made impressions early on that good skin and teeth were the foundations to good health and beauty.

All of the interviewees, and again especially the youngest in the study, were concerned about the impact the environment can have on the health of their skin. Sun blocks and products with high levels of SPF were more on their minds then ever before. For some the point of entry in skin care more than anything else was sun protection.

One universal issue among all of the interviewees was confusion over which products to use. The conversations often lead to skepticism that many of the products offered with new ingredients or benefits were just marketing efforts to get women to buy more products. As one of the interviewees remarked, "If the product was advertised as new and improved a year ago, why do they need to announce that they the same product has been improved again within a year"?

In asking women to be more specific about the Olay versus the L'Oreal skincare products there was a clear distinction between the two brands.

The L'Oreal Paris skincare portfolio raised concerns among the women interviewed because of the number of products in the line up and their "scientific" nature. With the first concern over the number of products, the interviewees found it difficult to determine which was best for them.

"I find that there are too many products. It is all too confusing. What's the difference between them? How would the average consumer figure this all out? It is not like a department store where there is someone there to explain it to you."

In addition to the confusion over the number of products was the number of "benefits" that the products were now offering.

"With all these benefits it makes you wonder if it's just another way to bring in new consumers. I understand the need to design something for the youth market but there are so many serums and creams. How many do you need? You just need a cleanser, toner and moisturizer. Too much stuff."

The second criticism in comparing L'Oreal Paris to Olay was that the L'Oreal Paris skin care was perceived as more chemical and scientific than Olay. The example used here was L'Oreal's Youth Code where women were either confused or very skeptical about the "genetic" aspect of the skincare line. In addition, the word "Youth" in the product name lead them to an impression that the product was for younger women.

"I don't buy it. I think the whole innovation thing is just to sell news. They tap into concerns to make it seem new. I like the tried and true, or natural. In six months there will be a new innovation. New products every six months is weird."

There was a lot of concern among the women regarding the product's genetic references.

"I think it is way too scientific for a beauty product. Sometimes I can't even get a shampoo to work. I would be a little worried about what this would do to me."

The concern over product action was coupled with its name.

"Youth Code sounds like something for my daughter."

As one women stated, "With this type of technology why isn't it a department store brand"?

"A formula to maintain your youth? I am skeptical about the genetic part. Is it a new thing or is it something they made up? More expensive brands would be using it."

Among the interviewees in the study who shopped at mass, L'Oreal Paris skincare was seen as a bit too scientific and perhaps containing chemical ingredients that these interviewees had concerns about. For some of the interviewees, especially those who purchased their skin care in department stores, the ingredients provided a reason to believe the product would actually "do something". However even these interviewees said that they would need to know more about the "effect" the chemicals in the product would have on their skin before considering purchasing.

" I used to use Revitalift but switched to Olay because I thought it [L'Oreal Paris] was too chemical, too scientific."

L'Oreal Paris was consistently associated with a more chemical based product.

"I don't know what it does [collagen], people have it injected, how can a cream do the same thing?"

This concern was mentioned across all of the L'Oreal skin care product lines.

"This is all too confusing, so much stuff written on these products, you need a medical dictionary to understand all this stuff."

In contrast to the interviewee's feelings towards L'Oreal Paris skincare was their take on Olay. First it is important to note that the Olay brands longevity in skincare provides a degree of trust and credibility that the L'Oreal Paris brand lacked. This thought was stated by most of the interviewees in the study.

Mentioned quite often by the interviewees was the fact that Olay has been around a long time. Many referenced that their mothers had used the brand in the course of the interviews on skin care. The brands longevity and heritage was never perceived as a brand that was out of date or touch with the interviewee's needs.

"I am familiar with both Olay and L'Oreal and I use Regenerist. My mom uses this and she looks good at fifty which is why I use it too."

It was not uncommon for the interviewees to reference their mother and their use of the Olay product line.

"I use Olay. My mom used it so that is how I started. I like Olay because it is only about skin care."

In the end the interviewees who were aware of both Olay and L'Oreal products viewed Olay as a more gentle approach to skin care. I think the important element here is that it is a brand that women referred to as a brand that cared about skin rather then a brand that was only about anti-aging.

The key driver within the Olay portfolio among women interviewed was the Regenerist line. Most women were familiar and had tried or were using this product line. The Definity line from Olay had a lower awareness among the women, but was seen as a good solution for skin discoloration or "aging spots'. In probing the ProX line the interviewees had mixed feelings about the use of the Olay name in association with this product.

For background, Olay launched Olay Professional ProX as a more premium skin care line. It was Procter & Gamble's attempt to enter a higher price point within the mass marketing of skin care and capitalized on what industry experts were calling the new "mass-tique", (prestige or department store inspired products at mass) segment forming. This new segment was now providing better quality at higher prices in mass outlets. The belief was that as women begin to trade up these products would be available. In addition to women trading up at mass was the strategy to target department store shoppers that were seeking quality products at a lower price point.

In its effort to be more premium and add greater skin care credibility Proctor & Gamble placed the ProX advertising in a scientific or clinical setting featuring scientists responsible for the skin care advancement. To further support an image of quality and superiority, the ProX price point hovered on the lower end of department store brands like Estee Lauder, creating a more expensive skin care option in mass market stores like Walmart.

For the most part the Olay name added credibility to the ProX among mass shoppers and had the opposite effect for those women who shopped in department stores. The reason is that in mass the Olay name added a degree of credibility, in department stores it cheapened the image.

The question of "professional" in the product name raised both negative and positives among the interviewees. The negative was that it was there to justify a higher price point in addition to raising skepticism on the idea of P&G professionals being the "experts" in skincare. On the plus side, the "professional" added the expectation of better product performance. The following quote from one of the interviewees summed up how the majority of the women in the study felt about ProX.

"This is what is so frustrating about skin care, it makes sense that it is more expensive [ProX] but it becomes so hard to choose because you don't know what you are really getting. I think it would work better because it is more expensive. Olay association is good in Walmart but if I saw ProX alone I would expect to see it at Saks."

There are three elements that separate the skincare consumer in regard to mass and department stores: price, education, and loyalty. This is not to say that there aren't various degrees for all three at mass, however, when we are talking about what influences women most in this segment at mass, it would be price and information. Loyalty is lower on the spectrum and women said they would "try" another brand if they had a coupon that made it worth their while.

The key discoveries about skin care from the interviewees in the groups were pretty black and white. If you were a department store user you wouldn't consider using a mass skin care brand. If you were a mass skin care brand user your loyalty was tied to cost and any beauty cream costing up to $25 dollars had better work.

Between the two companies, L'Oreal Paris and Olay, most of the interviewees in the study thought of L'Oreal as a "shampoo, color and cosmetic" company and had little awareness of their skin care line. The company has historically been know for hair color and hair care making it more challenging for the other segments to be noticed. Conversely Olay's heritage and longevity is a double edge sword for women. It's either a "not for me brand given that my mother used it" or on the positive side of things, "it must be good since it has been around forever".

Across the board the interviewees felt that if the brand expected them to "pay more" then the brand better be able to explain what it really will do. The department store women had a bit less skepticism given how they learned about products via "one-on-one service experiences in high end store like Saks". To that point, women who shopped mass admitted to going into a department store, when they could, to find out more about a particular product or ingredient then shop for something similar at mass.

One important discovery was that celebrity had very little rec-ognition across the brands. Perhaps this was the result of Olay at the time having none (as mentioned earlier they are now they are featuring Katie Holmes), and, L'Oreal having a number of celebri-ties for skin care segmented by age. Of all of those associated with L'Oreal Paris it was Andie MacDowell and Diane Keaton who were mentioned and well liked among the interviewees.

I think the two significant insights learned in talking to the inter-viewees was the growing concern over ingredient and its ultimate effect on ones chemistry. Here interviewees were beginning to pre-scribe to a less is more approach to doing too much and looking for alternate products with a more natural base. The interviewees expressed their concern about chemicals, especially those that they couldn't even pronounce, being absorbed into their bodies. This growing concern played nicely into the second, and for me the most important insight, in regard to women and skin care.

Most of the interviewees in the study, both young and old, felt that holding on to ones youth wasn't of great importance in their lives. Yes they all admitted to wanting to look youthful, but not necessarily "young". This notion of "eternal youth" was some-thing that was for "some Hollywood starlet" or "trophy wife". The feeling of "that's not for me" resonated across all demograph-ics within the study. A recent essay, "A Prize That's a Slap in the Face", written by Roxanne Roberts for the Style section of The Washington Post expands further on the topic of skin care prod-ucts and aging.

The writer expresses her frustration over More Magazine's, a lifestyle magazine targeted to women forty plus, decision to run a contest called "Women with More". The objective of the contest was to celebrate the personal accomplishments of its readers. The prize for the first three hundred entries was a bottle of ROC Retinol Correxion Deep Wrinkle Serum. The grand prize for four lucky ladies was a trip to New York for a photo shoot and a complete Roc Skincare package.

So why did Ms. Roberts have and issue with the prize? I believe that Roxanne Roberts tapped into how many women feel today about aging. As she wrote in her essay, "A magazine dedicated to celebrating the complex lives of mature professional women thinks that the best way to honor them is to help them try to look younger". She believes that it is all part of "The schizophrenic reality of women and aging".

When asked about their decision to reward women with wrinkle cream, More Magazine's editor noted the perfect alignment between the publication and Roc Skincare. Jeannie Shao Collins stated, "The brand perfectly aligns with the magazine's goal of celebrating confident, successful and beautiful women, both inside and out". She goes on to say the products are "dedicated to enhancing women's confidence as they age".

Most people would agree that looking good at any age is a reasonable goal. What Roxanne Roberts adamantly disagrees with is a magazine, whose average female reader is forty-eight, would reward women of personal achievement with a wrinkle cream. Her point reinforced what many women in the study had said about skin care and looking good for your age, versus the desire to look young. Or as Ms. Roberts wrote, "That the best way to age is to not look old".

In general, the women interviewed were consistent with three aspects when it came to skin care in their lives. Of course efficacy and cost was the universal consideration but after that there was the concern that chemical ingredients may not be a good thing in the long term. Next, expressed mainly among the "Boomer" interviewees who felt that age and youth were being redefined by their generation. They were less concerned about staying young and becoming more "comfortable in their own skin". The thought that was consistently voiced by them was that it was less important to look young and more important to look good for their age. This thought was once expressed in a slogan for Olay, "Love the skin you're in". Perhaps given what some of the interviewees said it's not a bad idea to return to it.

Does She or Doesn't She?

T he question often asked by beauty companies about celebrities is does she or doesn't she add any value? Given the number of celebrities that represent beauty products one can assume that "she does". So, the next question would be "How?"

Let's start with what defines celebrity. A celebrity is defined as a person who has a prominent profile in day-to-day media and because of this commands some degree of public fascination and influence. A celebrity is usually expected to be wealthy (commonly denoted as a person with *fame and fortune*), endowed with great popular appeal, prominence in a particular field, and is easily recognized by the general public.

The key words in this definition are <u>influence</u>, <u>popular appeal</u> and <u>easily recognizable</u>. Those words sum up the value a celebrity can provide any brand. Now, add to it personal style, beauty and charisma, the celebrity becomes the beauty ambassador for the brand.

While women do have difficulty with matching celebrity to brands you must realize that among the major mass beauty brands sold in the US which include L'Oreal Paris, Revlon, Cover Girl, Neutrogena, the majority, with the exception of Maybelline, use celebrity women on a regular basis. Maybelline has from time to time featured Christy Turlington, who is known for being part of the super model era and representing Calvin Klein for almost twenty years.

There are approximately thirty female celebrities that represent the major mass beauty brands in the US. These brands also represent nearly seventy-five percent of the total beauty sales that is approximately forty billion dollars in the US market. Some of them have represented multiple brands along the way. Take for example Julianne Moore who signed on as a Revlon Spokesperson in 2002 and was contracted to L'Oreal Paris in 2012. Kerry Washington, once a spokeswoman for L'Oreal Paris signed up in 2013 to be the "new face" of Neutrogena. As a Cover Girl in the 60's, and the Clairol spokeswoman in the 70's, Cybil Sheppard ended her commercial beauty reign with L'Oreal Preference Hair Color in the early 90's. She remained the "All American blonde" along the way.

Thinking back to the time when I was involved with beauty advertising I had worked with a number of well-known celebrities. I knew that if I were to do anything with this newfound Avon connection, it wouldn't be like the good old days sipping a cappuccino with Jenifer Lopez on location for a shampoo commercial.

It was her first L'Oreal Paris commercial and she talked about how proud she was to be the first Latina woman to represent the brand. It was late 1997 and up until that time Jennifer was famous for her break out role in the movie *Selena* that had debuted that same year. Not only was she the first Latina spokesperson for L'Oreal Paris, she was also the first Latina actress to earn over one million dollars for her performance in *Out of Sight* starring opposite George Clooney the following year.

From the moment I met Jennifer I was enchanted by her cool style, open demeanor, and natural beauty. At the time, she possessed a wide-eyed innocence that was magnetic. During that first production she invited me, and a few others, to her first husband Ojni Noa's LA restaurant the Conga Club. It was the last time we had the opportunity to casually hang out. Six months after that first shoot she changed management. Given her trajectory to stardom it was understandable. (And, within a year after that night at the Conga Club, she and Ojni split and spent a decade in court fighting over the right to her photos and videos). All I can say is "...but they seemed so happy at the time".

Moving from United Artist to another agency JLO was now under the watchful eye of high power music moguls and behind the scene there was PDiddy/Sean Combs... It was all in the timing as her debut CD *On the 6* was being released and her new entourage being formed. Her entourage was known to be the biggest in Hollywood at the time (who was counting?) and it seemed that way to everyone watching.

There were a few more productions with Jennifer each becoming more challenging than the last. This was as a result of her mega-star stature and the ever-growing protective circle that surrounded her. It was a fascinating experience for me to watch. I had met many a celebrity like Heather Locklear by this time in my career along with those that would become celebrities like Amanda Seyfried, but never had the opportunity to witness a megastar in the making until I met Jennifer Lopez.

My first celebrity shoot was with Vidal Sassoon in 1986. The world renowned hair stylist, famous for creating the first geometric cut in the 60's, was in New York to shoot a commercial for the hair care line named after him and now owned by Proctor & Gamble. Three words that I would use to describe him are elegant, soft-spoken, and spiritual. He had an aura around him even on the set that created a calm in the midst of production chaos. His passion and creativity changed the way the world looked at hair. I witnessed that same passion when he spoke to the camera and said the words, "If you don't look good, we don't look good".

One last celebrity moment was my first meeting Diane Keaton at the Polo Lounge in Beverly Hills back in 2006. I was awestruck not only by her presence but the setting as well. When she arrived we were seated at a very discrete outdoor banquette table. The setting was ultra Hollywood, and while people met there for lunch, they also met there to see who else was in the place. The world seems to be divided between those who find Diane Keaton a cutting edge fashionista, and those who think her wardrobe is over-stylized and over-the-top. So I was careful to note every detail of her wardrobe the day we met. Diane enters wearing a black silk skirt that was puffed out and cinched at the waist by a wide black leather belt. Black leggings led to black oxford loafers. She wore a top that resembled a man's white cotton button down only more fitted with an open neck and a long pointed collar. With sunglasses on she stepped over to the table. Wearing a white wool felt bowler hat she smiled and said "Hi, I'm Diane".

Celebrity for beauty brands can be expensive. While the numbers and terms are unique to each one, the same industry of agents and lawyers have a good idea of what celebrity X is making on a particular brand, or what brand X is offering a particular celebrity to sign. This can sometimes cause a bidding war between brands. Obviously certain beauty brands have more cache than others and the beauty segment often has a lot to do with the celebrity's choice. A twenty-five year old starlet would have to think twice about doing an anti-aging skin care advertisement. For that matter so would a forty-five year old that's concerned about protecting her youthful image in the Hollywood market.

The negotiations of many of these contracts can become contentious. With the spirit on both sides of "let's see how much we can get", in the end it all depends on how much each side wants the relationship to happen. The bigger the celebrity the larger the package, which starts with money and ends with a set number of workdays allowed. Generally speaking, the bigger the star, the fewer the days available given their intense schedules. Then, of course, there are the "requests" of each celebrity. This doesn't apply to all but, in my experience I got to see a lot. From the size of the celebrity entourage that traveled first class or, in some cases, by private jet from coast to coast, to the trainer, masseuse or nutritionist, required to be on set. I've even witnessed a Shaman blessing the location at the request of the celebrity. Keep in mind that most of the contracts provide for an 8 to 10 hour workday and the clock would start ticking upon pick up at the celebs home or hotel. You prayed that there would be little traffic.

Once on set there would be a myriad of issues beginning with getting a group from both the agency and client to agree on which outfit to present to the celebrity for fear that if the celebrity went through the wardrobe or 'rack', as it is called, we might end up with something that was not a first or second choice. (I know you are wondering why a sweep of the rejects weren't removed and the answer is that a smart celebrity knows that trick so in the end it would only amount to a waste of time).

When the celebrity, who in my experience always had the last word, approves the wardrobe one hopes that the others in the general beauty assembly (creative directors and clients) agree. If not, and after some conversation, a plan to deal with it in post-production—change the color, neck line, skirt length, or recreate something entirely different is generally offered up by a qualified producer as a possible option. This helps to save time and money with the hope that the celebrity doesn't have final approval for the advertising, which again depends on how big a star she is and if she has the last word, it may buy some time to get her to change her mind.

Next is hair and make-up artists, or the 'vanity team', as they are referred to. The celebrity generally chooses this team and more often is part of her own team. The reason for this and quite understandably, it is her image that needs to be protected. The wrong shade of a Tangerine Sorbet lipstick has the potential of hurting a beauty image especially in today's social sharing world.

For most of us this was the group (make up and hair experts) to get close to. They were in the know and knew how to approach the celebrity while at the same time being very protective. While the clock was ticking on the eight-hour day, generally three to four hours are spent in hair and make-up then at about this time, a break for a one-hour lunch (union requirement) is called leaving sometimes only three hours to shoot a commercial.

With that time-ticking challenge in mind, there were occasions when a celebrity who had reviewed the script in advance of the shooting day decides on set they are not happy with it. Keep in mind that most of the celebrities have a "final script or creative approval" written into their contracts. Given this authority a production could be delayed for script revisions if the celebrity had not taken time to provide comments prior to the shoot. Even worse than that, they do not want to say anything on camera that makes it appear that they are trying to sell something. This situation generally occurs towards the end of the make-up process and just before the first take on set is to happen. At this point, a very experienced producer, writer, account director, or therapist is called in to negotiate a resolution that will be acceptable to the beauty client. Sometimes it is a quick fix, sometimes not. I recall one occasion when the celebrity refused to mention the name of the product! (It's okay. She hasn't been back on TV since her last show was cancelled).

With all of this and the fact that there is such confusion matching celebrity to brands, one would ask the question 'why do it?' The simple answer is because the right celebrity matched up to the right brand can create magic. They can make a brand instantly popular or make a tired brand look totally fresh and modern again. A celebrity can make a brand top of mind for a consumer overnight. If it is the right fit, the celebrity becomes the face, attitude and voice of the brand.

Building awareness is what a celebrity can help a brand do immediately. The more well known the celebrity is, the more impact she provides. It is especially powerful when the celebrity is unexpected and can provide news value as in the case of Ellen Degeneres and Cover Girl. Not only is Ellen extremely popular, she provides for Cover Girl the added advantage of being a real make over as she is not known for glamour or being 'made up'. Ellen's beauty transformation is credible and provides living proof of the product benefits.

Credibility is what all brands need in order to succeed with women. If the celebrity does not provide credibility, then it's unlikely her association with a brand will influence a woman to consider purchasing. The beauty world is wrought with skepticism and given to exaggerated promises and benefits. For example the very thought of looking ten years younger after one week of applying an anti-aging product could only be possible if it came with a scalpel and a qualified plastic surgeon, or if you think you can go from dark brown to platinum blonde without using bleach think again. Add in a celebrity that lacks credibility in regard to actually using or applying the product and the brand has a problem.

If the woman has the slightest doubt that the celebrity being featured never even touched the product then there is no credibility that the product would deliver on its promise. The majority of the interviewees I spoke with found it hard to believe that these Hollywood ladies are using mass brands and, if they are, it is because they are being paid to as underscored by the following quotes:

"It depends on the way the celebrity looks, but we all know that there isn't a lot of credibility behind it with them using a stylist or makeup person to put it together for them."

"The first thing that I think of is how much money did they receive to do the commercial."

Certain celebrities do provide both the awareness and credibility and were mentioned by a few of our women.

"Comes down to credibility, like, I don't think Drew Barrymore used Cover Girl, but I believe that Andie MacDowell does use L'Oreal. "

With celebrity and credibility comes the challenge of diversity. While Revlon was the first, Cover Girl followed quickly in the early 90's signing Lena Ogilvie, an African American model. This led to the onboarding, albeit it all to slow, of most of the major beauty brands to follow the trend.

The beauty brands that I have mentioned have developed a portfolio of diverse celebrities. Women today are greatly influenced by a celebrity that shares physical characteristics with them. Latina women, like all women, want to see how celebrities with their coloration look wearing the beauty product advertised. An Asian American can no longer relate or even be influenced by the "All American blonde". She is looking for the celebrity that looks most like her for inspiration knowing that she will never look like Gwen Stefani with a deep red lip. Those companies that incorporate diversity into their celebrity portfolio will appeal best to the evolving ethnic communities across the country. Women today are looking at beauty brands with a far more critical eye. Now it is all about personalization and "what works for me".

Among some of the women, there was a credibility factor when it came to mass brands and well know celebrities. One interviewee, referencing a past L'Oreal Casting Crème Hair Color commercial, questioned whether or not a famous person like Penelope Cruz would really use a home hair-coloring product when she has "her own people to do it." The skepticism around celebrity and product usage, especially mass beauty brands, was consistent among most of the interviewees in the study. The women did not believe that they would get the same look or result as the celebrity without the same expertise provided by makeup and hair professionals. The one thing that the interviewees all agreed on was that the celebrity brought value to a product by creating an awareness of the brand despite having some difficulty matching celebrity to brands and product. I think the following quotes from three of the women interviewed represents the sentiment of the group.

"I was never into the celebrity thing in school. Whoever is in the advertising would not influence my decision. I notice the celebrity, but there are way too many and it is confusing."

"Celebrities provide impact, makes you aware but doesn't make me want to buy. When I saw Sarah Jessica Parker do a commercial, I noticed it, but I didn't buy it."

"I think they help to get the brand noticed, but there is always the question of whether or not they use the products. I think it is more credible when they do infomercials like the one Claire Danes did for eyelashes [Latisse]."

When looking at beauty brands in the mass market, celebrity plays an important role. The celebrity's presence in advertising can make a difference and depending on her stature she can elevate a brand's image overnight. While the interviewees in the study did not feel the celebrity was a deciding factor to their purchasing, they did admit to being influenced by a celebrity. "It got me to notice", was generally the feeling and for a beauty brand, being noticed is one of the most important elements. In the business it is called 'building awareness'.

Women shopping for mass brands need more education, which is provided in the advertising since there is little to no counter help available in store. Prestige brands, although even this is beginning to change, don't require layers of copy in their ads since women can get information at the store counter. That department store consumer relies on the sales person to inform her on the what, why, and how to use a product or regime. Overtime, this often leads to a relationship that is as important to the shopper as seeing her own therapist. Less layering in the advertising allowed for great visual impact and a more prestigious image.

The differences in the way celebrities are used in mass brand advertising versus department or prestige is enormous. This holds true for both TV and magazine advertising. The department store brands are generally the 'designer' brands in beauty. For example, Chanel cosmetics need very little introduction for those purchasing beauty products at that price point. Generally speaking, an advertisement for Chanel would most likely include the prestige packaging, a beautiful red lip color on a celebrity like Natalie Portman and the Chanel logo. Now, if we were to compare this to L'Oreal Paris advertising for lipstick, we would see those elements and more. The more would include 'before and after' illustrations of the product benefit (e.g., moisturization or long lasting), plus additional copy that would provide an explanation of why it's better, newer or different. A mass beauty brand needs to communicate more information in advertising because they do not have the in-store sales support compared to department store brands. As a result, in the advertising, the celebrity for a mass-market brand is sharing her portrait with product demos, bottle and a lot more copy. The result is a dilution of the celebrity's impact while increasing the brands 'message' or product explanation. This reality is a big factor in why some celebrities would not consider contracts with mass brands knowing that the 'sell' factor can influence their own image. For many celebrities their personal brand image outweighs the image of any beauty brand. Scarlett Johansson's brief relationship with L'Oreal Paris in 2006 is a prime example of this. She was not interested in "selling" product. She preferred to be the beauty icon of a brand. She moved on within a couple of years to become the face of Dolce & Gabbana. (Good luck with that.)

Authenticity is a crucial element to drive connection between the celebrity and the audience. It is different than credibility in that it is driven by a visual element in the example of 'does she really color her own hair with a box product from Kmart?' Authenticity for a celebrity is closely linked to the words she speaks on camera. For example, would it feel authentic to have Diane Keaton talk about the Hyaluronic Acid contained in L'Oreal Paris skin care products? (No.)

Many of the women that I spoke with referred to this as the "real" factor. Without looking at any commercials, the interviewees recalled commercials where certain celebrities seemed to be saying things that "real" people would never say. They seemed to be referring to things like ingredients that were "weird" or "something I never heard of". The second part of this was if the celebrity appeared "too done" making her "realness" questionable. Yes, women do have higher expectations for celebrities because they continue to look to them for inspiration, but if it is pushed too far it can be a complete turn off. When authenticity is part of the message, women respond positively.

Interviewees do agree that if a celebrity is used in an authentic way she can add value to the brand. This authenticity could come from mentoring other women about beauty products and talking about their personal discoveries when searching for solutions. Many of the interviewees referenced the Pro-Activ celebrities Jessica Simpson and Katy Perry as two celebrities who talked about their personal issue with acne and the positive results from the product.

"I like authenticity, a balance of the celebrity and the brand."

"Celebrities bring a lot to the package…it helps if the celebrity is normal without a lot of baggage."

The value even extended into being good role models for women, especially in the emerging world of beauty and diversity.

"Celebrities can be mentors for women like Jennifer Lopez is for younger women."

The ultimate connection/buy in for women is if they share something in common with the celebrity whether it's ethnicity, age, or physical characteristics in hair, or skin tone. This comment made by one of the interviewees supports this theory:

"I like seeing Jennifer Lopez wearing different cosmetics because she and I have similar skin tones. If the celebrity shares similarities with me then I would consider buying it."

Yet the celebrity game, while already a bit cluttered, is becoming even more so with a new form of influencer. The beauty blogger is quickly becoming the new celebrity.

The beauty blogger in this new digital age has the ability to reach millions of women and express her point of view on products. The bigger her following, the more amplification the message receives as a result of the social sharing that occurs. If she is credible and reviews a product favorably, it is as good as a best friend telling her it's a must have!

Who are these new celebrities and why do they have such influence? To begin with they can be anyone who likes to write about or in some cases video their experience with beauty products. The top video bloggers generally have some credentials either from being in fashion or styling, or are simply hard-core beauty junkies. In the past women seeking out information about products and "how to" would look to beauty magazines as their source for information. Women still do that but with the use of the Internet, they can cast a much wider net and obtain product information and on-line demonstration on how to apply and use various products. From eyeliner to hair coloring, the beauty bloggers are the new experts to guide you along the way.

The one very powerful difference between the traditional celebrity and the blogger celebrity is that the latter has instant credibility given the before and after demonstrations that she provides. The viewer sees her transform using the product without an expert stylist or a make up person performing the application for her. It's true that anyone can start a beauty blog but the ones that generally capture a large fan base or following are those that seem to be in the know about beauty. For women searching for answers they are the new source of information joining magazine beauty editors for the latest tips on product and application.

One of the first Video Bloggers on the beauty scene was Michelle Phan. Starting in 2005 Michelle used YouTube as a vehicle for her homemade beauty tutorials styled after Bob Ross, the American painter and host of the PBS program "The Joy of Painting". With the use of a voiceover while demonstrating how to get the look, she was one of the first bloggers to garner millions of followers. The onset of 'how to do it yourself' on YouTube has become the new in-store demonstration by an expert or sales person. The beauty of this is that it is 24/7 and in the privacy of your home.

Given the age of her audience, Phan introduced an entirely new and much younger consumer to Lancôme. Just by watching the application of selected Lancôme make up products being demon-strated online, a new generation of younger women discovered this department store brand primarily used by mature women.

From Beauty Bloggers to Red Carpet Celebrities, these are the ambassadors for beauty brands. Like the products they speak on behalf of, they are each unique in their own way. Their influence on women can vary depending on notoriety, likeability, credibility and authentic-ity. This collection of celebrity drives billions of dollars in annual sales with their ability to inspire and get women to spend money on the products they endorse. It is as simple as motivating a woman to try a new shade of lip color or inspiring another to go for a complete make over. Some of the celebrities mentioned have had successful long-term relationships with brands, as in the example of Andie MacDowell and L'Oreal Paris, making it difficult to think about one without the other.

At the end of the interviews on celebrity value it was clear that there is a positive influence on women when awareness, credibil-ity, and authenticity come together. This influence begins with the awareness a celebrity can bring to a product. This awareness can be one that is unexpected thus gets noticed as in the example of Pink for Cover Girl or it can be an alignment of images that are a perfect fit as in the case of Jennifer Lopez and L'Oreal Paris. Both provide value to building the awareness of the brand.

This awareness is only as good as the credibility of the celebrity look and performance. This is mainly driven by the belief that women have that the celebrity is actually using the products she is endorsing.

Finally, authenticity is key for women to believe in what the celebrity and, ultimately, the brand are saying. It simply comes down to the words used to express a feeling about the product; are they in the words of the celebrity or advertiser? Would a woman listening to a celebrity want to hear her drone on about the "advanced technology" or relay how she feels about the results? For the message to be truly relatable for other women, it requires that the celebrity come across in an authentic manner, expressing how she personally feels about the product experience and results.

Writing about celebrities and their relationship with brands and influence on consumers, I am reminded just how privileged I have been to be able to work with many talented, smart, passionate, and beautiful female celebrities during my association with L'Oreal Paris. What I have observed over the many years is the commonality they all embraced; a belief about all women. This belief was that every woman has value and should be reminded of it. Each of the celebrities personalized this message when it was their moment to express the sentiment using four words, "Because You're Worth It".

Women on Women

I n addition to the conversations around brand image, product innovation and celebrity value, I wanted to explore with the interviewees who they thought represented today's new beauty icon.

Over the centuries and around the world the beauty icon has been represented in art, theatre, movies and magazines. Historically, iconic women, such as Cleopatra and Josephine, with their captivating beauty and feminine mystique, have ruled empires.

In the 20's it was Louise Brooks, the 30's-Gretta Garbo, the 40's-Rita Hayworth, the 50's- Marilyn Monroe, the 60's-Twiggy, the 70's-Farrah Fawcett and on and on.

Over time beauty icons come and go while beauty companies are always on the look out for the next one. It has always been important to a beauty brand to discover the "new face" of beauty at least up until now according to the interviewees. In the past this iconic beauty would be the inspiration for other women to try a product or beauty look. Today the term beauty icon is being redefined. The beauty icon is becoming a life icon admired for more then her physical attributes-redefining how other women influence women. The interviewees in the study across all age groups defined the new beauty icon as someone of accomplishment with strength and personal style.

The modern beauty icon is a woman that is far more dimensional than even ten years ago. The women in the study look up to other women who go beyond setting beauty trends to women who contribute to society. This new icon is more than a beauty symbol-she inspires a type of evolved lifestyle. An example of this is Oprah whose celebrity goes beyond movies and television. As a global icon her influence on women extends into politics and philanthropy. To the interviewees in the study she is a perfect representation of a modern day beauty icon.

The interviewees were well aware of the changing world of influencers in beauty and ironically it was not all about Hollywood celebrities. Many of the women referred to women in politics as the new icons with the belief that iconic beauty goes further than a woman's physical attributes. To the interviewees it is about "style and power." Hillary Clinton and Michelle Obama were the two women mostly mentioned here. This was the perfect combination of influencing characteristics according to the interviewees. The women interviewed were more interested in what a women stands for rather then what she looks like. While in the past a woman's viewpoint on beauty and lifestyle may have had greater separation, the women interviewed saw the two intertwined in a more realistic way.

The women interviewed recognized the importance of beauty brands in their lives, but were clear about their role and relevance.

In this changing world the definition of beauty is part of that evolution. As part of this movement it was impossible for the interviewee to identify a singular beauty icon for today. The one that came closest was Angelina Jolie.

And even if there was one beauty icon, like Angelina Jolie, it's no longer just an endorsement from a beautiful celebrity that has the greatest influence on women. Today it is about cost and ingredients. These two elements according to the interviewees in the study are far more important to them than ever before.

The interviewees in the study did begin to answer the question of who today's beauty icon is, but it is not an easy answer to come by. Today's beauty icon is a fusion of many things that go beyond being beautiful. Intelligence, power and influence have been added to the beauty icon's criteria. What also became evident is how important diversity in the beauty world was to the interviewees. Women talked about the importance of individuality and their desire for beauty brands to understand their needs and speak to them with sincerity and respect.

"I think beauty will always be important. It will always evolve. It is becoming more relevant and purposeful as time goes on. Today it's not about one look or person it's all about personal expression."

Fin de Siècle

T he French have an expression, "fin de siècle", translated, it is the belief that when one cycle ends another begins. When I started this 'Ding Dong, Avon Calling' project I never thought I would end up writing a book about it. The truth is I was looking for a way to keep myself involved in the beauty world. It's been awhile since I made that decisive call to Human Resources to resign. The end of a cycle. But that call put me on the road to this valuable adventure-another cycle begins.

After finishing up with my interviews I ended my weekly relationship with Avon. I am back at the house in the country finishing this book. Instead of making tuna fish sandwiches in bare feet it's grilled cheese in warm slippers. The temperature outside is hovering around fifteen degrees. The "Global Appointment Kit" in English number 3463040 is sitting to my right (just to double check that I haven't missed something) and somewhere among the electronic clutter in my closet is the mini recorder that captured the interviews.

By now all of the products that I purchased for this experiment have been passed along to friends and family. It never disappoints me to see the expression of delight when a woman discovers that a gift bag is filled with beauty products. I listened to every taped interview again to verify emerging attitudes and beliefs about beauty companies, products and celebrities. The patterns were consistent and the greatest enjoyment beyond the insights discovered was in witnessing the delight women seemed to have when they could speak freely about what beauty means to them and ultimately what makes them feel beautiful. Being a good listener helped me along the way as well.

From the onset of this study there were a few specific points I wanted to discuss with women; brand impressions, product innovation, celebrity value and beauty reality.

Brand impressions for the women in this study were based on either personal experience or past references passed along from mother to daughter. With a diverse age group commenting on various brands, the images of the various brands were consistent among the interviewees. For example, Maybelline despite its efforts to become more sophisticated, still had the image of being a younger brand, "my first cosmetic". A brand like Revlon with its on-going reinvention was still perceived as "an old brand". The conclusion here is that a beauty brand with longevity requires greater effort to "evolve" and shift brand perceptions. A valuable insight about the mass-market consumer is that her brand impression is driven by her personal experience with one of its products. However, just because she is loyal to a particular brand of mascara doesn't mean she is going to purchase the same brand's skin care or shampoo.

Product innovation is very important in beauty according to the women in this study. Creating "better value for your money" and "makes it easier" were common themes when discussing product evaluation. This section of the interviews also highlighted the passion or criticism each woman was able to express with actual product in hand. The product benefit or packaging allowed for a more specific dialogue about the brand. In some cases it reinforced brand impressions, in others, shifted them. New packaging for Maybelline's Fit Me is a good example of shifting the brands image in a positive way. L'Oreal Paris's brand image was reinforced with the products used in the study as an industry leader in innovation.

Celebrity value is important for a brand to be recognized. However in the beauty world the proliferation of celebrities representing beauty companies is creating confusion. The women in this study understood the value of having a celebrity getting the brand noticed, but had difficulty matching the celebrity to the actual brand. In some cases if the celebrity did not have similar physical characteristic to the woman herself-blue eyes, dark skin, blonde hair-then the celebrity and the product weren't perceived as relevant. Another issue with celebrity was credibility. Many of the women in the study did not believe that a Hollywood star would be at home coloring her own hair or polishing her own nails.

Beauty reality is a catch all for many of the insights learned from the interviewees. From the Dove Real Beauty campaign discussion to today's new beauty icon, women are relating to beauty brands in a different manner. In the past women would follow beauty brands setting new trends. A great parody on this is a TV commercial for Yoplait GoGurt called "Mom's Smokey Eye". In this commercial a middle-aged mother is passing lunch bags to her two children who are shocked with the raccoon like eye make up mom is wearing. In a rather casual tone her response to their questionable expressions is "What? It's called a Smokey Eye".

Contributing to this nonconformist attitude about beauty, women are discovering alternate ways of self-expression that are replacing make up and hair color as the primary route to do so. For the younger generation body piercing and tattoos are the new beauty accessories. For the older generation of women in the study it is about self-acceptance. For the fifty plus generation it's not about looking younger, rather it is about looking good for your age. For some in this age group hair color requires too much maintenance so going naturally grey or white is a better option. Another insight on beauty reality provided by the interviewees is the need for greater diversification across the beauty brands. To be inspired, women need to see a reflection, both physical and emotional, of themselves in the brand messaging.

One final thought. On top of the Avon materials that were being stored away was one of the original orientation pamphlets, "Believe In Your Success". This makes me smile. Under that is the "Avon Beauty At Your Fingertips", one of the selling tools that promise to be helpful providing tips on conversation starters. The Avon selling tips are broken down into five steps that are meant as an aid when approaching a potential customer. They are:

1. Approach each sale and use these product information cards as a conversation starter.
2. Determine Customer's need, that's exactly the purpose of these cards.
3. Present product and use the information on these cards along with samples and demos
4. Answer questions and add your personal testimonials to the benefits mentioned on the product fact cards.
5. Close the sale going through the current brochure to find the products your customer has selected. Use special brochure offers to clinch the sale.

Now that I have completed this project I decided to revise these five steps to make them relevant in my life going forward.

1. Approach every opportunity you are given with genuine interest and passion.
2. Determine Customer's need by listening closely and you will understand a great deal more about people and what's going on around you.
3. Present products knowing that you are your own product so discover what benefit you can provide and go for it.
4. Answer questions directly and without any compromise.
5. Close the sale by exploring everything, but in the process strive to be an expert at one thing.

Finally a big thanks to all the women who were part of this project. I learned a great deal from each of you. We discussed perceptions and beliefs on the topics of beauty, products and celebrity that have provided insight and content for this book. More so we got to spend some time getting to know a little more about each other in the process - which for me was even more rewarding.

Glossary of Terms

Application tool   Brushes, sponges, rollers and even fingers are all considered application tools in beauty. They are used to apply product to the face and eyes. For lip, a doe tip sponge is often used for soft and even coverage. The term application tool is now being expanded to include the world of digital with beauty apps such as the "Makeup Genius App" from L'Oreal Paris.

Brand Equity   The brand power or value that is built over time in the minds of consumers. Strong brand equity allows a manufacturer to expand its product line under the same name. For example the brand equity of Apple is one of innovation, design and exceptional user (consumer) experience upon which they continue to introduce new products.

Class of trade   Class of trade in manufacturing refers to four areas of retail; Department store, Mass outlet, Food and Drug. An example of each respectively would be Saks/Bloomingdales, Walmart/Kmart, Pathmark/Kroger, and CVS/Rite Aid.

Concept development   In marketing/advertising this is the practice of developing ideas into simple communication elements that are then exposed to people for feedback. It is commonly used to measure the interest level for the idea.

Creative execution   The skill of an art director and copywriter is to take an idea or concept and execute it on paper/computer. It is part of the process of bringing ideas to life. The creative execution traditionally was either in print or film. Today it is expanded into the social and digital space that provides for greater exposure/amplification of the idea.

Discovery phase   This term is commonly used in research and development. It is a fact-gathering phase in the process. Elements included in this are establishing the project objective, critical success factors, defining the scope of the project, best practices evaluation and initial planning. The goal is to collect enough data to begin concept development leading to creative execution of ideas.

Focus group

A form of qualitative research in which people are asked about their opinions, perceptions, and attitudes towards an idea, product, service, concept, advertisement, or packaging.

Gibson Girl

Image created by illustrator Charles Gibson. She embodied the ideal woman of the early 1900's. "With her hair piled atop her head and a waist so tiny as to defy belief, the Gibson Girl represented a serene self-confidence that could surmount any problem". This ideal woman became the standard in beauty suggesting a new female independence with one of privilege and glamour.

Masstique

In the beauty world this is the merging of department store or prestige value with mass-market cost. This relatively new term is applied to beauty brands that offer similar prestige value/performance at mass brand prices. It is a strong trend in skin This relatively new term is applied to beauty brands that offer similar prestige value/performance at mass brand prices. It is a strong trend in skin care with expressions like "why pay more for a department store brand when this one for a fraction of the cost will do the same?"

Mindscape   A mental landscape or that which remains in the mind. Memories from experience of place, people and things you have done.

Product awareness   Similar to brand awareness, this is the degree to which a product is recognized by people, especially its intended target. Product awareness is an important measurement in determining advertising effectiveness.

Product descriptors   The communication of what a product does, mostly its benefit and form. It is a way to position a product intention. It is often used to announce new technology including form, liquid, gel or spray.

Product stability   The ability of a product to remain stable or unchanged in its composition due to a variety of conditions. These conditions can include, temperature, altitude, shock, humidity and time. Testing for product stability is essential for new formulas prior to introduction and launch.

Price point

The suggested retail price of a product in store. Price points are generally determined by cost of goods, profit margin and competitive activity. Price points in beauty sometimes are higher to provide an "impression" that the product is superior to its competition.

Retail relationship

This is the relationship that is shared between manufacturer and retailer. In the beauty world it is a vital relationship given the increased competition for shelf space in store. This "retail real estate" as it is called is an important element for beauty companies to maintain in order to sustain existing lines of products while they launch new ones. This relationship can also help to provide intelligence on what the competition is planning to do with new product launches down the road.

Sample Audience

A selection of people that resemble a brands target audience. For example a sample of women between the ages of 16 and 60 who use beauty products on a regular basis would be a typical sample for large beauty care companies.

Superiority claims Generally a statistic used in advertising to convince that one product is better than another. Examples include claims like "makes hair 10 times stronger than the leading shampoo" and "97% of women who tried saw visible results in 2 weeks". Superiority claims must be supported in order for them to be used in communications. The FDA and/or competition often challenge them if they seem to be too far fetched.

Store Check A practice used by most manufacturers to inspect their products and the retail environment. What a manufacturer looks for during a store check is product placement, distribution, out of stock issues, signage, competitive presence and overall store appearance.

Voice Over The unseen person or announcer used to narrate a commercial, movie or broadcast. Voice over talent is often chosen based on their voice characteristic matching up with that of the brand.

Made in the USA
Middletown, DE
30 September 2015